THE LIGHTNING STICK

BOOKS BY THE AUTHOR

Women of the Apache Nation: Voices of Truth

Survival of the Spirit: Chiricahua Apaches in Captivity

*Medicine Women, Curanderas, and Women Doctors
(with Bobette Perrone and Victoria Krueger)*

THE LIGHTNING STICK

ARROWS, WOUNDS, AND
INDIAN LEGENDS

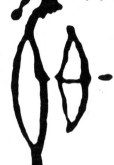

H. HENRIETTA STOCKEL

UNIVERSITY OF NEVADA PRESS
RENO, LAS VEGAS, LONDON

The paper used in this book meets the requirements of American
National Standard for Information Sciences—Permanence of Paper
for Printed Library Materials, ANSI Z39.48-1984. Binding
materials were selected for strength and durability.

Library of Congress Cataloging-in-Publication Data
Stockel, H. Henrietta, 1938–
    The lightning stick: arrows, wounds, and Indian legends
  / H. Henrietta Stockel.
      p. cm. —
    Includes bibliographical references and index.
    ISBN 0-87417-266-7 (paper : acid free paper)
    1. Surgery, Military—Southwest, New—History—19th
century. 2. Bow and arrow—Southwest, New—History—19th
century. 3. Stab wounds. 4. Indian weapons—North
America. I. Title.
RD201.S76   1995
617.1'43—dc20   94-43926
                                              CIP

University of Nevada Press, Reno, Nevada 89557 USA
Copyright © 1995 by University of Nevada Press
All rights reserved
The Lightning Stick is the University of Nevada Press's
first book to be composed in-house.
Typeface: Century Old Style, using Aldus PageMaker.
Book design by Heather Goulding
Jacket design by Erin Kirk New
Printed in the United States of America

9 8 7 6 5 4 3 2 1

To Dan L. Thrapp,
whose wise counsel
and friendship will remain
with me for the rest of my life.

May the Great Spirit
guide and protect you,
wherever you are.

"Who killed Cock Robin?"
"I," said the sparrow,
"With my bow and arrow,
I killed Cock Robin."
"Who saw him die?"
"I," said the fly,
"With my little eye,
I saw him die."

—Mother Goose

CONTENTS

ACKNOWLEDGMENTS

I love this book. Which is not to say that I didn't love the others I have written or will not love the books I plan for the future. But this one is special. Maybe it's because of the sheer folly of writing about arrow wounds as the world approaches the millennium wrapped in the potential for planetary nuclear destruction. Maybe it's because Western scientific medicine has doubled and redoubled on itself so many times that what was fresh and new five years ago is obsolete today. And maybe it's because people usually don't die from arrow wounds anymore. Today, late in the twentieth century, children are shot in city streets as they jump rope on the filthy sidewalks, the victims of snipers shooting at someone else. At least the wars on the frontier were fought *for* something, regardless of which side one supported. Now, America fights wars in foreign countries to ensure access to oil or to make sure the correct dictator remains in power even while the "enemy" burns the very same oil.

This little book may reflect my wish to return to less complex times, or it may be a tribute to the Native Americans who so desperately defended their homelands with bows and arrows. Then again, it may honor the wounded men of the U.S. Army of the West, or it may show my respect for the physicians who risked their own lives and limbs to treat the soldiers' injuries. Or it may just be something else and therefore none of the above.

Whatever it is, my pal Louise d'Avignon Fairchild is a big part of it, and I thank her over and over again for everything. Most especially do I appreciate her listening to my frustrations and complaints during the course of writing this book when I was unable to get to the computer for days on end when beautiful sentences were burning holes in my head. I thank two superb and loving physicians, Simon Dack and Lillian Batlin, who were so much a part of my younger life and whose natural kindness, incredible medical skills, and bald-faced need to alleviate suffering instilled in me a lifelong interest in all things medical. I thank my friends for the quizzical looks on their faces and the questions in their voices whenever I mention this book. Hard as it might be for them to believe, I have taken a brief vacation from writing about the Chiricahua Apaches—and that seems very strange indeed to the people who know me best. However, readers will recognize my abiding interest in the Chiricahuas from my various references throughout the text.

Many of the staff at the University of New Mexico Health Sciences Center Library provided me with information, photos and slides of skulls, catchy phrases, ideas, and rich written material. *Gracias*.

One very sad but important note. I want to honor, pay tribute to, and particularly thank respected writer and historian Dan L. Thrapp, who died shortly after reviewing this manuscript. Dan guided and encouraged me in all of my writing through the last several years, and it feels strange to be suddenly "alone," to know that he no longer lives just down the road in Tucson. I know that Dan, and the late author Eve Ball, will continue to inspire me as I become more immersed in what is now my life's work: writing about the historical American West and Southwest and its people. My home. My heart.

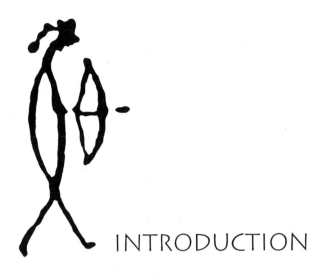

INTRODUCTION

It's a simple and obvious truth that American military men and women no longer go off to war fearing fatal injuries from bows and arrows. Weaponry now is quite different—much more technologically advanced, if you will—and once-deadly arrowheads are now popular collectors' items. But not so long ago the soldiers who formed the U.S. Army must have been exceedingly brave to confront Native Americans armed with these "primitive weapons." Primitive or not, the folks who made and used bows and arrows meant business.

The Indian group known as the Tonto Apaches, for example, carried arrows that were three feet long from notch to point. The arrows were made from a particular cane that grew in the Arizona mountains around springs and other sources of water. About six inches from the notch, the cane shaft was winged with four strips of feathers held in place by threads of sinew, probably stripped from a deer's leg. At the opposite end of the arrow, the Tonto Apaches preferred a colored point, "as if with the blood of some animal,"[1] made of quartz, flint, or, occasionally, iron. The arrowhead was sharp at the point and slightly serrated, all the better to tear into an enemy's flesh. It has been said that "primitive man became a mineralogist almost with the first use of unworked stones" because of the need to consider the quality—the toughness and sharpness—of the stones he selected for his arrow-

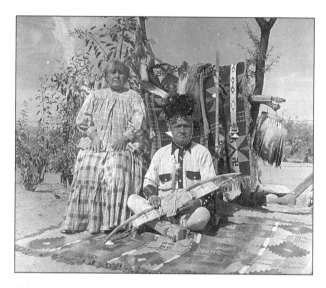

San Carlos Apache leader Shorty Delmar and wife, ca. 1935, probably on the San Carlos Apache Reservation in Arizona. Delmar holding bow and quiver full of arrows. (Photo by Margaret McKittrich; courtesy Museum of New Mexico, #41839)

heads.[2] The color of the arrowheads was also important to several tribes that associated certain hues with the spirit world. Through trial and error, early humans learned which materials were most effective and thus began to discriminate among the types of stones readily available for use as arrowheads.

The bow used by the natives of the desert and mountain Southwest was probably constructed of a wood similar to mulberry or reed. It was about five feet long and strengthened by sinew, which was wrapped around strategic sections. It was straight for the most part, but curved slightly toward its extremities. The ready availability of straight woods meant that members of southwestern tribes spent less time working on each arrow than did some of their counterparts in other regions of the continent. Even then, time was valuable, especially when tribes were preparing for warfare, and the natural shape of the raw wood used for arrows added considerably to a group's readiness for battle.

A bow and arrow had to be lethal, no matter what the tribe of its user, and all the techniques used to construct the weapon were designed to ensure maximum injury to the recipient. Further, the soldiers who chased Apaches and others probably didn't realize that warriors frequently blessed their weapons prior to battle as well. Whether or not the ancient rituals actually added to the weapon's efficiency depended on the individual's perspective and adherence to cultural customs. The efficacy of this spiritual enhancement would no doubt have been endorsed by most Indians and disregarded by most non-Indians. Whatever their individual beliefs, soldiers and others in the line of fire (including Indians at war with other tribes) knew that to be superficially wounded by an arrow was bad enough, but a more serious injury could be fatal.

Those who did not die immediately from the wound itself often suffered from complications. Wildfire infections caused by arrow wounds brought an agonizing death. The Indians, at least, could seek spiritual surcease in the form of culturally sanctioned ceremonies. Although many injured soldiers undoubtedly prayed, the white culture had no healing rites specifically conducted to alleviate the pain and suffering of war wounds. In contrast, when a Pima Indian was injured in battle (or fell ill from an ailment not related to warfare), a native healer destroyed the sickness "by shooting painted arrows from painted bows at imaginary evil spirits supposed to be hovering in the vicinity of the patient."[3] Whether this tribal remedy actually aided recovery might be questioned by many, but quite a few native healers still defend the ancient paths toward healing. And the psychological effects of strong belief in a system of healing must not be underestimated.

The military and civilian enforcers of the westward expansion of the United States, and others, were not always face-to-face with the frightening circumstances of battle, of course. Soldiers and settlers in the American West and Southwest worried about, handled, and confronted other, less threatening matters as well, as is evident from their diaries, journals, church records, and so on. The routine of daily living usually takes second place to the more exciting, more flamboyant side of life, however, especially insofar as the old West is concerned. So in retrospect, it appears that battles always raged, that innocent people always died, that Indians always lost, and that blood always ran.

Much of the current interest in cowboys and Indians, running now at full throttle, started in 1990 with Kevin Costner's epic motion picture, *Dances with Wolves*. After that, it was a good bet that Geronimo, the old Chiricahua Apache bugaboo who haunts America's history, would make another appearance, as he does from time to time in the media and in popular literature. Sure enough, in the early 1990s Geronimo was the focus of a major motion picture and a television "special"—shown simultaneously. Each film purports to show the "human" side of the famous warrior, but both fall short.[4] Depictions will fail, to greater or lesser extents, until the history is written by the vanquished instead of the victors. And, as a nation, we are a long way from allowing that to happen.[5]

Nonetheless, it is the records of the conquerors and their heirs, personal and professional, that I have relied on here to create, or re-create, certain situations and circumstances of the old West—arrow wounds in particular. Even though the odds were against them, many men and women recuperated from their wounds, and without antibiotics. These survivors were fortunate because surprisingly adequate medical techniques and implements had been developed to deal with arrow wounds. In many cases a stone, iron, or wooden arrowhead embedded in tissue or bone could be yanked out or pulled through, bleeding could be controlled, the gaping hole could be cleaned and dressed, and the aftereffects anticipated.

The arrowheads used by Native Americans—against each other and against the newcomers—occasionally carried poisons, but they really didn't need to. The Indians were such skilled bowmen that any enhancement to the basics was normally unnecessary. In dipping their arrowheads into venom, vegetable poisons, and putrid animal matter, however, Native Americans joined a long tradition of acceptable warfare practices.[6] The actual toxic effect of "poison-tipped" arrows has always been overplayed by Hollywood, so much so that contaminated arrowheads have become an essential ingredient in the collective consciousness of the West. Such is the power of the modern media. This sophisticated nuclear-age society has evolved to a point, certainly insofar as a retrospective look at the American frontier is concerned, where the truth diminishes the folklore.

There are relatively few instances in which the legends of a people—their folklore, so to speak—were directly communicated to outsiders without embellishment. One such example is the material disclosed by Ishi, "the last wild Indian in America."[7] The only survivor of the Yahi tribe in California, Ishi simply walked out of his homeland on August 29, 1911, and became an incomparable informant. His remarkable tale has captured the imagination of historians, anthropologists, students of Native American studies, writers, and people everywhere who have heard it.

Although all the information Ishi conveyed during his very few years among white people (he died of tuberculosis, a disease he acquired after entering white society, on March 25, 1916) is important and certainly essential to an understanding of the Yahis' cultural customs, his descriptions of the construction of his bow, arrows, and arrowheads are of special interest to me.

Saxton Pope's writings about Ishi's traditional methods of making weapons remain among the classic literature on the subject.[8] Pope recorded quite a bit about Ishi, including the Yahi name for a bow, *man-nee*, which Ishi said was usually a short, flat piece of mountain juniper or incense cedar backed with sinew. Ishi acquired the wood by splitting a limb from a tree and using the outer layers after scraping the wood with flint or rubbing it on sandstone. He recurved the bow by bending the wood backward over a heated stone, and he seasoned it for months or years by placing it in a dark, dry place. After seasoning, the bow was strengthened with sinew. First Ishi made a glue by boiling salmon skin and applying it to the roughened back of the bow. Then he took strips of sinew made from deer leg tendons, 8 to 14 inches long, and laid them on the bow, carefully covering the entire back of the bow very thickly. At the nocks he added a circular binding of the same organic material. Then the bow was permitted to season in the sun for several weeks. The completed bow was usually about 44 inches long, 0.6 by 1.5 inches at the handle, 0.6 by 1.9 inches at midlimb, and 0.3 by 0.75 inch at the nock. It pulled about forty pounds.

While the bow was seasoning, Ishi made the bowstring, or *chalman'i*, from the outer group of tendons in a deer's shank. These he tore free from their muscle bundles with his teeth, then he chewed the mass apart into threads as thick as dental floss. If the tendons were dry instead of fresh, Ishi soaked them in warm water before putting them in his mouth. He spun a string by fixing one end of a bundle of tendons to a stationary point and twisting the other end between his fingers, adding more and more threads of tendon to the cord. Eventually the *chalman'i* became a very tight, simple twist an eighth of an inch thick and about five feet long. He then attached the

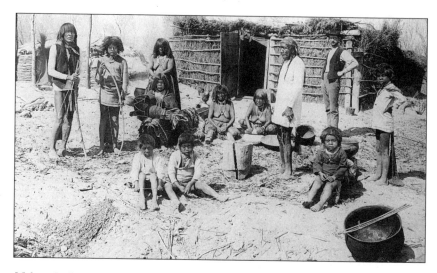

Mohave Indian camp in California, ca. 1883. Note men at left holding bows and arrows and arrows resting on black iron pot at lower right. (Photo by Ben Wittick; courtesy School of American Research Collections, Museum of New Mexico, #16339)

opposite end to another fixed point and let the bowstring dry. According to Robert F. Heizer and Theodora Kroeber, its final diameter was about a tenth of an inch.[9]

When initially stringing the bow, Ishi sat down and placed the upper nock behind his left heel, the belly toward him, the handle against his right knee, and the lower limb upward in his left hand. He wound the string twice around the nock, turned backward and wound in the opposite direction for several laps, then fixed the end with a couple of slipknots.

Next, Ishi addressed the arrows, or *sawa*. For these the Yahi used several kinds of wood; Ishi's favorite was hazelwood. He selected the straightest shoots of hazel, cut them about a yard long, and then stripped the bark with his thumbnail. The length of a Yahi hunting arrow was 29 inches, its diameter at the middle was 0.3 inch, and the total weight was 300 grains. Ishi usually made them in groups of five, then selected the best and bound them together with a cord. The bundles were allowed to season for periods ranging from one week to a year. Using a little stick as a paintbrush, Ishi liked to paint the arrows in his favorite colors of green and red, which he obtained by mixing plant pigments with gum or sap from trees. "When the paint was dry," reported Heizer and Kroeber, "he ran a broad ring of glue above and below it, at the site of the subsequent binding which holds the feathers."[10]

Ishi preferred eagle feathers for his arrows but often had to settle for donations from hawks, owls, wild geese, herons, quail, pigeons, turkeys, and blue jays. Frequently buzzard wings provided the four-inch-long feathers that Ishi affixcd to his arrows. With a sharp piece of obsidian, he cut three plumes from the same wing for each arrow, using a straight stick as a guide and laying the arrow on a flat piece of wood. Ishi collected the feathers in groups of three and soaked them in warm water until they were soft. Then he bound them down with deer tendon that he had chewed to a pulp and pulled out of his mouth in long strings.

For points, called *pana k'aina,* Ishi preferred flint or obsidian for hunting. The Yahis used blunt arrows for target practice. Most tribes were very frugal with their arrowheads, using them only in the hunt or during warfare. Tips for Yahi arrows were made only after the proper ceremony had been performed. Before beginning, the arrow maker smeared his face with mud and sat in a quiet, secluded place, usually on a hot day. He took a chunk of obsidian and smashed it on another rock to cause several small pieces to flake off. With a thick piece of buckskin protecting the palm of his left hand, the man placed one of the pieces of obsidian flat on the buckskin. Holding a deer antler in his right hand, he pressed the point of the antler against the edge of the piece of obsidian so that glass flew off from the pressure. The designer continued shaping the stone, turning it over and over, until an acceptable arrowhead resulted. Yahi points were generally about 2 inches long, 0.9 inch wide, and 0.1 inch thick. After the points were set in place on the end of the arrow shaft with heated resin and bound with sinew, a Yahi warrior was ready to hunt or fight.

From time to time bits of the obsidian flakes would fly into the eyes of the arrowhead maker, who followed a careful procedure to remove them. First, he pulled down his lower eyelid with the left forefinger, being careful not to blink or rub the lid. Bending over, he then thumped himself on the crown of his head with his right hand. The blow usually was enough to dislodge any foreign body from the eye.

Ishi carried five to sixty arrows in his quiver, which was made of otter skin with the fur side turned out and the hair running upward. Ishi's quiver was 34 inches long, 8 inches wide at the upper end, and 4 inches wide at the lower end. The entire otter skin was used to make the quiver. The skin was completely removed from the otter's body except for an incision over the buttocks. The hind legs were split and left dangling, and the forelegs became two sheaths of skin inverted inside the quiver. The otter's mouth was sewn shut with tendon, and the split tail became the carrying strap.[11] Ishi also carried his bow in the quiver, and extra arrowheads and sinew were carried in a little bag. When he was actively shooting, he tucked several arrows under his right arm, which he kept close to his side while drawing the bow.

Pope, who had watched Ishi use his bow, concluded that Ishi was not a good target shooter, but he did think that Ishi probably "could excel the white man" when shooting game.[12] Obviously, Pope had a low opinion of non-Indian archers. He had other strong views as well. In skilled hands, he thought, whether they be native or non-native, the arrow was more merciful to man and beast than was the bullet. "An arrow wound," he wrote,

> is clean-cut and the hemorrhage is tremendous, but if not im-
> mediately fatal it heals readily and does little harm. The pain is
> not greater with the arrow than with the bullet. . . . And those
> who think the bullet is more certain and humane than the ar-
> row have no accurate knowledge on which to base their com-
> parison. Our experience has proved the contrary to be the case.
> Yet we [shoot the bow] because we love it . . . it is an emotion
> difficult to explain.[13]

So, then, is this why I have written a book about arrow wounds and other calamities? Because I too love the bow and arrow? The answer, like the answers to all important questions in life, is subjective and depends on many variables. First of all, a complete understanding of the westward expansion movement is impossible without considering the topic of weaponry. Second, and strangely, the bow and arrow has not received the attention it merits. Arrows were deadly in native-against-native encounters, but they were no match for the lightning-fast bullets shot across the land with malice by both Indian and non-Indian in later years. And perhaps that is why bows and arrows, and arrow wounds in general, have not been addressed in more detail by historians, scholars, and writers. By the same token, might there come a time when the literature on ammunition and guns as we know them will be replaced by extensive writings about, say, atomic and nuclear weapons used by individuals for offensive and defensive purposes? Maybe so.

Speaking for myself, however, I have become aware lately that bows and arrows are still in use, and I don't mean as exhibits in museums or objets d'art or hunters' weapons. More and more, it seems, I read or hear about deadly or harmful incidents caused, purposely or not, by these weapons. And then I think back to a totally different era in American history, one still enshrouded in myth and, perhaps because of the commotion kicked up by so many swirling legends, greatly misunderstood. A "little" book about arrow wounds won't dispel the dust totally, of course, but perhaps it might help those of us who are traditionalists, and others standing on the lip of a new century, to reflect on how far we as a people have come during just the last 150 years in developing deadly weapons of war—and wondering where the next millennium will take us.

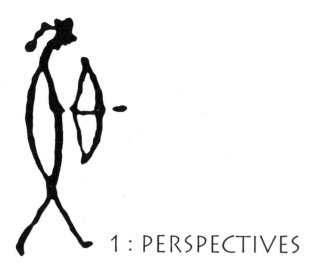

1 : PERSPECTIVES

The topic of arrow wounds and similar calamities that occurred more than a century ago seems anachronistic and out of place in contemporary society. After all, humankind is poised and ready to greet a new millennium—the twenty-first century. Why in the world would anyone want to go *backward* in time? Well, quite a few modern men and women of a particular generation could probably be coaxed into admitting an enduring personal interest in bows and arrows, perhaps begun in darkened movie theaters when they were children. The Saturday afternoon shoot-'em-ups held sway over millions of youngsters in the 1940s and 1950s and created in many an affinity with the cowboys and Indians of the old West. Others may have become acquainted with bows and arrows when they studied world history in junior high or high school and heard about the exploits of the ferocious Attila the Hun—who, by the way, used a bow with stiffened ears set at a sharply recurved angle, a form that allowed Attila and the members of his horde to bend heavier bows with less effort. They could fire from horseback and penetrate the armor worn by their enemies. By the time the Huns used the bow and arrow, however, it was already an ancient weapon, its origins obscured in murky antiquity.

Edward McEwen, Robert L. Miller, and Christopher A. Bergman traced the origins of the bow and arrow from Paleolithic times through the seventeenth century in Europe and Asia. In an article published in

Scientific American, the three concluded that "bows display important and practical variations in construction, ranging from designs barely more than branches with strings attached to what can only be described as sophisticated mechanical devices."[1] The article describes the basic design of the bow as a two-armed spring, spanned and held under tension by a string. The pressure increases when the bowstring is drawn back, and when the bowstring is released, the energy is transferred to the arrow, throwing it into flight. Modifications on that fundamental concept were made down across the millennia, and the bow and arrow developed into an efficient instrument for hunting and combat.

Early Asian bowyers were particular about all the materials that went into the construction of their bows, but they were especially concerned with the adhesive supplements, derived from hide and fish swim bladders, that they glued to the back of the bow. This technique allowed them to shorten the bow without a concomitant loss of draw length or risk of breakage. The smaller, stronger bows thus created were easier to handle on horseback and more efficient. (Long, heavy bow limbs use a great deal of energy as they move forward with the release of the string, thus reducing the energy available to be transferred to the projectile.)

The ancient knowledge that a bow's action can actually be enhanced by shortening it and adding strengthening substances such as sinew may have been carried into the New World by the migrating adventurers who came to be known as Native Americans. In any case, the Plains tribes—the Sioux and the Comanche—centuries after the Asians and in a markedly different location, developed bows with the same architecture, and they applied the same raw organic materials to improve their weapons' performance. And they didn't stop there: "Many tribes later removed the wood entirely, substituting elk antler or mountain sheep horn for the wood belly—a development only one stage away from a true composite bow."[2]

The complex bow was also used by Asian horsemen, who, in addition to adding sinew, glued water buffalo horns to their bows' bellies to further strengthen the weapon and cause it to snap back to its original shape after being pulled. According to the *Scientific American* article by McEwen, Miller, and Bergman, the Asian angular bow is one of the earliest surviving examples of the composite bow, which may have first appeared during the third millennium B.C. Illustrations of this weapon nearly two thousand years old appear on Mesopotamian seals, Assyrian monumental reliefs, and Egyptian tomb paintings. King Tutankhamen's tomb contained thirty-two angular composite bows, fourteen wooden self-bows, and 430 arrows, as well as quivers and bow cases.

The bow in its many variations reigned supreme until the sixteenth century, when the invention and widespread distribution of firearms completely overshadowed it. Among some peoples, however, including the indigenous occupants of North America, the bow and arrow long remained the most effective missile-firing agent available to hunters and warriors.

In 1882, United States Army surgeon J. H. Bill expressed his fascination with the bow: "From its infancy, the human race has drawn the bow. Accordingly, we find that the arrow [is] of particular interest to surgeons."[3] And certainly on the frontier, mighty warriors like Geronimo, the infamous Chiricahua Apache, and others could always resort to deadly bows and arrows when their supply of guns and ammunition was exhausted.[4]

Even now, bows and arrows are still used as instruments of war in some spots on the globe. As recently as 1986, for example, the *Los Angeles Times* reported clashes with spears, stones, and bows and arrows between members of the Jiga tribe of Papua—New Guinea and a rival group. About three thousand tribesmen fought in hand-to-hand combat in the provincial capital of Mount Hagan, a battle brought on when a funeral procession broke up into a bloody riot. One person was killed, a large number were injured, and several shops, banks, and government offices were damaged before police used tear gas to end the mayhem. About eighty people were arrested, but only two were charged and jailed for rioting. Only outsiders, it seemed, became excited over the incident. "We fight. We settle. It is our way and we are happy. It always works," said Nelson Wale, a young man of twenty-one years with a deep scar on his forehead.[5]

An even more recent example of one modern fellow's use of the bow and arrow was reported by the Associated Press in May 1993. Anthony Roberts, a young man living in Portland, Oregon, was shot through the head with an arrow by a friend, according to the news report. This was not, as might first be imagined, a fight over a girlfriend or rival gang members seeking revenge. On the contrary, the accident occurred during an initiation ritual into a rafting and outdoor group called Mountain Men Anonymous. Both Roberts and his buddy had been drinking before the archer aimed his bow at a gallon can balanced on his pal's head. The arrow's tip went eight to ten inches into Roberts's brain, slicing through soft facial tissue a fraction of an inch away from major blood vessels. Although he survived, the unemployed carpenter lost his right eye, possibly ruining forever his dream of entering the fraternity of mountain men. On the other hand, Roberts's fearless but foolish attempt to pull the arrow out of his head during the helicopter ride to the hospital could earn him a lifetime membership in the club. Fortunately for Roberts, paramedics on the flight restrained him. Doctors later drilled a large hole around the arrow's tip at the back of his skull, then pulled the arrow through and out. "I really feel stupid," said the sober and chastened would-be mountain man at a press conference about ten days after the surgery.[6]

A more deadly use of a bow and arrows fatally wounded Ken Kirkman, an Albuquerque, New Mexico, businessman. Kirkman's son Jason pumped three big-game-hunting bladed arrows into his sleeping father after a domestic dispute. An autopsy revealed that one of the arrows had penetrated under the right rib cage, one was embedded in the right shoulder, and the third had lodged in the right biceps. From the angle of the arrows, officials speculated that Kirkman bolted upright after the first arrow struck his chest and then was hit the second and third times. The arrows carried metal points just above cones studded with razorlike blades.[7]

Putting aside malevolent uses of the weapon, another New Mexico story, this one about bowyer Harold Groves, demonstrates a unique and more positive use of a bow and arrows. Groves, now more than seventy years old, recalled being part of a famous project back in the 1940s, when archery was his favorite hobby. In those days his regular job was as a machinist in Los Alamos, New Mexico, where scientists were busy designing and building the bomb that changed the history of the world. For recreation, the atomic wizards constructed a bow on paper and claimed it was better than any in existence. Knowing of Groves's interest and talent, they approached him with their blueprints, and he followed through and built it. "They were Oppenheimer and those others, so I tried it," he said modestly. The first time he shot the new bow, Groves broke the world distance record. The machinist continued to better all statistics, even his own, until he quit long-distance shooting in 1966 because "those heavy bows were tearing up my shoulders." His record of shooting a hunting arrow 444 yards still stands.[8]

Groves became a part of American history when he helped Los Alamos engineers build a bridge across an abyss that separated the laboratory from the town. Responding to a request from management, Groves shot arrows trailing lines from one side of the canyon to the other. These lines subsequently hauled heavier cables across, allowing the engineers to start construction. On that windy mesa near Los Alamos, Harold Groves unwittingly joined more than two sides of a huge fracture in the earth. With his accurate marksmanship, his arrows married the past to the future and the primitive to the sophisticated. Harold Groves connected the bow and arrow to the atom bomb for all time.

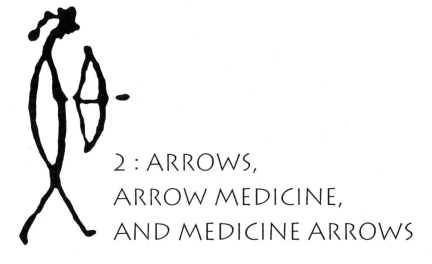

2 : ARROWS,
ARROW MEDICINE,
AND MEDICINE ARROWS

When all the universe was still black and the sun had not yet been created, when there were no stars, no plants, no trees, no people, no animals, *something* caused a change. Whatever happened, that monumental event found form not only in the physical world as we know it but also in stories of the creation—ways to explain it. These tales about the Beginning, usually called creation myths, form the center of every culture's system of beliefs. They make things plausible; they satisfy; they interpret.[1] They are not necessarily logical and they don't have to be alike, but all have been handed down from the elders; all go back to the time before time.[2]

Down through the ages, orally communicated cultural knowledge has been essential to preserving identity, customs, and beliefs. Now that oral history is acknowledged as a legitimate academic tool, diverse cultural groups worldwide are having their origins and other important occurrences documented by researchers—and rightfully so, for the power of legends should not be underestimated.

The Old Testament myth of Adam and Eve in the Garden of Eden, for example, forms one of the bases of a religion that has lasted five or six thousand years. It matters not whether the adventures in Paradise are true or false, whether they were written in the Bible as fact, allegory, or metaphor, or whether they can be scientifically proved or disproved. Adam and Eve have mightily influenced the course of events on this planet.

Native American creation myths have no biblical foundation (although a few mention a great flood) and often are dissimilar from one tribe to the next. In some cases contradictory versions coexist within a single cultural circle. Nevertheless, the more traditional tribes commonly rely on these tales to explain eternal mysteries. For example, while one creation myth may describe the world before the start of time when no human beings were yet alive,[3] another may describe its people as being "descended from the sun."[4]

Geronimo told one version of the Chiricahua Apache creation myth that describes a great battle between the birds and the beasts.[5] The beasts were armed with clubs, but a great bird, the eagle, shared with the Apaches his bow and arrows and even taught them how to use the weapon. After the war was over and the birds were victorious, only a few human beings were still alive. One of them was White Painted Woman. Years later she bore a son whom she hid in a cave lest the one beast remaining alive, a dragon, should find and devour her beloved boy. The feared disaster almost happened, but the youngster defeated the dragon with a bow and arrows, and he was then named Apache. The almighty Giver of Life, called Ussen by the Apache people, taught the boy how to prepare herbs for medicine, how to hunt, and how to fight. Thereafter, the youngster wore eagle feathers as a sign of justice, wisdom, and power.

According to this legend the Chiricahuas derive their heritage through bows and arrows given to them in antiquity by none other than their Creator, who chose the eagle as his messenger. Additionally, this weapon is said to have saved the life of one of the culture's most revered deities—White Painted Woman. In this particular creation myth, the Apaches are alive today because of her son's skill with the weapon. Thus, the power and the symbolism of bows and arrows within the Chiricahua Apache culture flow from their Creator and other supernatural beings. Knowing that, it becomes easier to understand an Apache's fierce commitment and willingness to die in battle, bow and arrows in hand.

A Seminole creation myth from 1824 also mentions bows and arrows. A chief of the Seminoles reported that

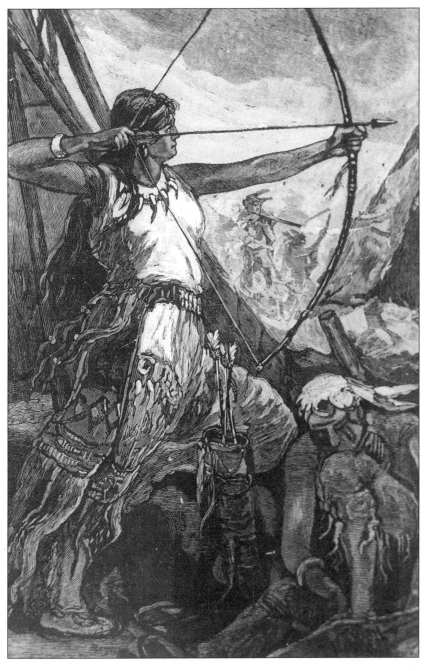

"Heroism of a Woman of the Nez Perces," 1898. Drawing by F. S. Church. Note the quiver with arrows near her left knee. (Courtesy Museum of New Mexico, #107725)

according to Indian traditions, the world was created by the Great Spirit; . . . he formed three men, an Indian, a white, and a black man; the Indian was the most perfect: they were called into his presence, and directed to select their employments; the Indian chose a bow and arrow, the white man a book, and the negro a spade.[6]

Legends other than creation myths also refer to bows and arrows. The weapons and their owners described in these tales provide role models for future warriors. For example, there is a Navajo story about a family's oldest son who "had made a long bow and lots of fine arrows with eagle feathers on them and he could sure shoot. . . . He could hit whatever he wanted to. His bow and arrows, his moccasins and his ability to run were exceptional." It is easy to imagine a young boy being inspired by this description and wanting to imitate a warrior whose unmatched aim, skill, and athletic ability are remembered forever. Another Navajo tale describes

a very big man [who] had a bow about four inches wide and about two inches thick; it was almost straight so the string was against it. He wore a big wrist guard. His arrows went so fast that as far as those stones (forty yards) you couldn't see them. He went to fight the Utes and he shot the leader right through the shield and the arrow went about that far (one and one-half inches) into his side and he went a little ways and then he died. The Utes all ran. When the leader is killed there is nothing else to do, you don't know what to do.[7]

This myth honors size and strength, which led to victory in battle thanks to the combination of man and arrows. Again, a story such as this one might influence a youngster in a manner that ultimately could benefit the tribe as a whole.

The Navajos respect the power of arrowheads, for they believe an arrowhead can do harm without being attached to a shaft or shot from a bow. One old tale tells of two men who demanded a fat sheep from a third; when the latter refused, the angry and spiteful men rode their horses to a high point overlooking the sheep's grazing area. Plotting revenge, "they put an arrowhead on a rock pointing to where that man lived. They fixed the arrowhead so it was tipping and was just about to fall. Then they prayed and did some things." The sheep rancher got word of what was happening and

> got a medicineman to make a bundle to protect his sheep. About two days later his daughter was out herding sheep and she saw the tracks of a bear. She went home and told the medicineman that those tracks went across her sheep on the east. He said, "That is good because the bear passed between the sheep and that arrowhead and that breaks the power" [of the evil sent outward from the arrowhead].[8]

The sheep were never harmed.

The Cheyenne of the northern Great Plains believe that the Big Dipper was created as a result of a situation involving a bow and arrows.[9] They tell of a girl who dyed porcupine quills to decorate the buffalo hides that her people wore. When she had made seven shirts, she left home to find her seven brothers, who had moved to the north. Dogs went along with her for protection, and she promised her mother that she would send them back as a sign that she had found her brothers. Carrying the shirts, the girl walked with her dogs for many days until she met her brothers and then sent the animals back home. Soon afterward, an entire herd of buffalo charged at the small group, who climbed a tree for safety. The largest buffalo continually butted the tree trunk with his massive head, using such force that the branches shook wildly. The frightened family knew that the tree couldn't withstand the blows for long, so the youngest brother, clad in the quill shirt his sister had made, aimed his bow and arrow toward the sun and let the arrow fly.

> Just as the tree was splitting in two, the girl and her seven brothers flew after the arrow. Glistening in their quillwork shirts, they floated right up to the sky, never to fall back down among the buffalo. There you can still see them on a clear night in the northern sky. The girl became the North Star. Around her turn the seven stars we call the Big Dipper. We see them there just as the Cheyenne Indians saw them long, long ago.[10]

Before bows and arrows appeared on the scene, Native Americans used spears to hunt and fight. Not much information relevant to

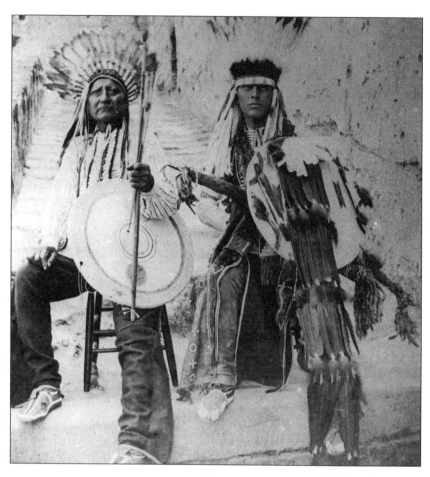

Cheyenne Chief Minimac (left) and his son Howling Wolf as prisoners of war in Fort Marion, Florida, ca. 1871–75. (Courtesy Museum of New Mexico, #70549)

these earlier weapons exists; the topic of spears with dartlike points is generally avoided in creation myths. Nonetheless, a rare find was made in California in 1793: an atlatl (rhymes with *battle*), a "fore-shafted dart with bone barb and flint point, sinew-backed bow, and double bladed paddle."[11] Some similar darts were found during a separate excavation south of that spot, in a cave in Baja California. They were bundled together and lying beside the skeleton of their owner, which was still fairly well preserved although hundreds of years old. Sketches show that these instruments actually resemble a spear, and they are extremely valuable for the glimpse they give into a time thought lost to history.[12]

According to William Massey, atlatls

vanished from the cultural inventory of [Baja California] between 1534 and 1643, shortly after the arrival of Europeans. Apparently, the dart thrower [as the weapon is called] was on the verge of disappearance. It is fortunate that the Spanish observed the survival.[13]

Not only did the Europeans witness atlatls in use, they also left written records of the weaponry used by the natives of Baja California. Many of the reports date back to the years between 1535 and 1697, before the geographical area was turned over to the Jesuits, and contain descriptive material on the use of the weapon and its construction.[14]

One of the earliest notations is from a document of the Cardona Company, which was permitted by the Spanish government to fish in the Gulf of California. Company ships under the command of Juan de Iturbe sailed to Baja California in 1615 and 1616. When he returned, Iturbe apparently told the owners about the indigenous peoples he encountered there. Subsequently, Nicholas de Cardona, one of the owners, wrote about the natives. Their weapons, he said, were "shafts inserted in a stick of two palms [in length], which, when they are thrown, go more rapidly than an arrow." A second account was written by Don Luis Cestín de Cañas, the governor of Sinaloa, who wrote about the neighboring Baja natives: "They also use some fire-hardened darts, which they throw with an instrument, with which they make them fly like an arrow."[15]

That the climate favors preservation in certain areas of California is indicated by the discovery in the 1940s of a complete Serrano arrow hidden beside some pack rat debris in a small vertical crevice of a large granite outcropping.[16] Found in San Bernardino County, this arrow is unusual just because it was in perfect condition when it was found. No other related remains were located with it. Since the arrow was within the territory previously occupied by Serrano Indians, it is assumed the weapon belonged to that ancient group of natives.

The Serrano arrow is composed of three parts: a cane shaft, a hardwood foreshaft, and a stone point of white chert. The overall length is 800 millimeters (31.4 inches), and the shaft diameter is 9 millimeters. A 7-millimeter-deep parallel-sided notch is cut at the base to receive the bowstring, with the end trimmed to form a broad V outline. The nock is cylindrical. Just beyond and crowding over the nock are three feathers, split down the quill: two from a western red-tailed hawk and the other from an adult pallid horned owl. The distal end shows three cut marks where the cane was trimmed to receive the hardwood insert. The foreshaft is held in place by thin pieces of wrapped sinew for a distance of 34 millimeters. On the main shaft, about midway in the wrapped section, a black band about 9 millimeters wide can be seen through the sinew. Just below the sinew wrapping holding the arrowhead on the foreshaft are two dark bands about 3 millimeters wide and 3 millimeters apart. A few other dark splotches occur at irregular intervals along the wooden shaft, possibly the remnants of similar bands.

X-rays of the Serrano arrow show the stone point being held in place by a sticky substance reinforced by the wrapping, which was applied in an X pattern. The glue was probably from a one-leaf piñon or creosote. The arrowhead itself is somewhat crudely flaked, with a concave base and slightly uneven side notching.[17]

Robert F. Heizer, discussing the skill required to shoot arrows such as the Serrano arrow described above, cited California's Shasta Indians as particularly skillful. His research revealed that in 1841 they could put up "a button at twenty yards distance, which one of them hit [with an arrow] three times out of five." Heizer also mentioned Indian marksmen who could "strike a ten-cent piece at a distance of twenty paces, six times out of ten" and those who could "hit a mark three inches in diameter at a distance of more than a hundred feet."[18]

Spanish explorers and other newcomers wrote in their journals about bows and arrows—and those who used them—from many tribes. Hernando de Soto, who explored the Mississippi River near Memphis in 1539–41, found that the natives were always ready for war and extremely skillful in battle:

> Before a Christian can make a single shot . . . an Indian will discharge three or four arrows; and he seldom misses. . . . Where the arrow meets with no armor, it pierces as deeply as the shaft from a crossbow. Their bows are very perfect; the arrows are made of certain canes, like reeds, very heavy, and so stiff that one of them, when sharpened, will pass through a target. Some

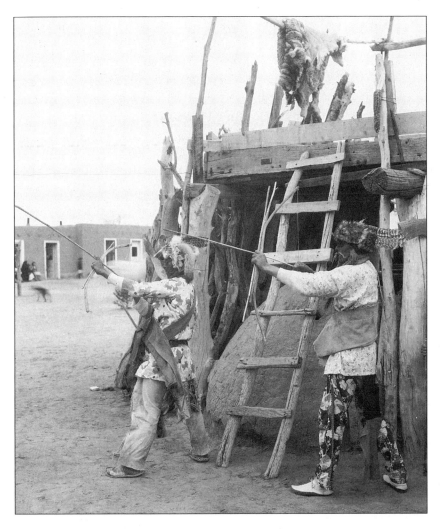

New Mexico's San Juan Pueblo Indians participating in a deer dance to ensure a good hunt, ca. 1935. (Photo by T. Harmon Parkhurst; courtesy Museum of New Mexico, #3852)

are pointed with the bone of a fish, sharp and like a chisel; others with some stone like a point of diamond; of such the greater number, when they strike upon armor, break at the place the parts are put together; . . . and will enter a shirt of mail, doing more injury than when armed.[19]

In 1538 Antonio de Espejo described the weapons of the Pueblo Indians of New Mexico: "Their arms consist of bows and arrows . . . ;

the arrows have fire-hardened shafts, the heads being of pointed flint, with which they easily pass through a coat of mail."[20] Apaches roaming the same area of the Southwest employed arrows about a foot long, crafted from a light rush or cane and bearing a point of iron, bone, or flint. "The Apaches shot their arrows with such force," reported D. E. Worcester, "that one would go through a man's body at 100 yards. . . . With this weapon an Apache was considered more than a match for any Spanish dragoon in single combat."[21]

Lieutenant Elliott Coues, an army doctor, arrived at Fort Whipple, near Prescott, Arizona, in 1864, when several bands of Apaches were raising havoc. He had many occasions to observe the clinical consequences of war against a powerful group of Indians, and he wrote about some of his experiences, particularly the extraction of Apache arrowheads from injured, dying, or dead soldiers:

> The heads were all of stone, quite small and sharp, and very brittle, so that they usually shivered when they struck a bone and the fragments were not easily removed. They were only held in place with gum in the shallow notch at the end of the small hardwood stick that was set in the large reed, and thus were always left in the wound when the stick was pulled out.

Dr. Coues believed that the Apaches poisoned the points of their arrowheads by dipping them in a deer's liver "into which a rattlesnake had been made to inject its venom, and which was then left to putrefy in the sun."[22] The Indians' use of viscera from all types of animals as the poisoning agent is the stuff of legends. One band of Apaches, the Lipans, dipped their arrows into the sap of the yucca, which they thought was very poisonous. According to the natives, the points of the yucca possess a mystic power that will adversely affect anyone hit by an arrow dipped in its sap.

The Comanches and Pawnees, who were very skilled bowmen, carried lances that resembled the atlatls of old—tips of swords (with no poison on them) inserted into wooden handles. From the middle of the 1700s onward the Comanches had firearms, but they continued to use bows and iron-tipped arrows when they shot from horseback, possibly because those weapons were noiseless and allowed the shooters to slip away from an ambush without revealing their location. In 1868, Richard J. Perry wrote that the bow and arrow in the hands of skillful warriors proves very deadly; it makes no noise and for night attacks or the taking off of sentinels, is far superior to the gun. Secondly, it is the best weapon that can be used in the chase, or, more properly, on the hunt, as half a dozen animals may be slain in a herd before their comrades are made aware of the fact. Thirdly, they are so light that they can be worn without the slightest sense of encumbrance. Fourthly, they can always be relied on, at close quarters, when other weapons fail, or ammunition, of which they possess limited supplies, gives out.[23]

Indians knew that the bullet supply was unpredictable but there was always abundant wood for arrows in the forests. As far back as the 1600s, Spaniard José Cortés wrote, "We can be sure that the reason why the Indians have not thrown away their bows and arrows when they manage to acquire a rifle is their frequent lack of ammunition and the total lack of means to repair them when they break down."[24] Along with the limited supply of ammunition and their stated inability to fix broken weapons, the natives' confidence in and steadfast use of bows and arrows had another dimension: healing.

Many tribes considered arrows to be sacred, a blessed gift from their Creator and the people's connection on earth with the supernatural. Traditional healers who incorporated arrows in healing rituals were particularly powerful, for they represented the Creator. In the Chemehuevi way, for example, an "arrow shaman" was a medicine man who could cure arrow wounds and some other injuries with "arrow medicine." He was stronger than many other medicine men and cured his patients "more rapidly than a regular shaman. He had no guardian spirit" because "he did not need one for he had a cool breath and a good hand." Although this medicine man "sang but two or three songs at a treatment, he dreamed many, beginning in early youth." To the Chemehuevi, the shaman's dreams of arrows and guns rendered both kinds of weapons

ineffectual as water. Arrow and bullet wounds, broken bones, and blows received from clubs, he treated chiefly by singing [the songs of his dreams] which braced the patient and overcame drowsiness. He also blew upon and pressed the body of the patient; he sucked only body wounds.

Arrow wounds were frequently worse than gunshot injuries because of the risk of infection caused by the difficulty in removing the arrowhead. On the other hand, there were many arrow doctors available to treat such injuries. One legend tells of a battle between two tribes, the Cocopa and the Yuma, in which two Yuma fighters were hurt. Fortunately, two Chemehuevi arrow doctors visiting the Yumas agreed to treat the unconscious and dying men. Obeying the medicine men's directions, the Yuma people cut down three or four willows to build a shade. In the evening one arrow doctor attended one of the young men and the other ministered to the second patient, both under the protection of the willow shade.

> They placed the warriors with their heads to the east. Then each doctor kicked the sand at the foot of his patient, then at the head. They started to sing and to blow their breaths upon the boys. They had finished four parts of the song and were blowing, when the boys opened their eyes. Each stood up, as though he had been asleep. The Yumas gave the doctors beads and other things in payment.[25]

While the introduction of firearms into Native American societies no doubt disrupted many an arrow shaman's specialized healing skills, other medicine men quickly adapted their ceremonies and practices to include injuries caused by guns. The Mohave Indians, for example, claim that in aboriginal times they possessed certain shamanistic practices that led to the cure of arrow wounds. After guns came into use, "they felt helpless, since arrow-wound magic could not cure gunshot wounds. The situation remained unsolved until a native shaman declared that he had received the power to cure gunshot wounds."[26] The tribe's emotional security was restored, and its social stability, which had been seriously disrupted when unfamiliar types of wounds were introduced into the community, returned. All it took was a declaration by the tribal healer that he had the power to cure bullet wounds.[27]

Well north of Mohave country, in America's northern Great Plains, Crow tribesmen were known for their aggressive, assertive behavior against other natives. Back in the days before Europeans moved into the area, a Crow warrior named Talks-with-the-Bear was very ill from an arrow wound. "In the group of buffalo hide tepees where his band is gathered for the summer hunt," wrote one physician,

> there is no one who has heard of the white man's medicine, for this is in the early nineteenth century when few white men live in Crow hunting country. The family of Talks-with-the-Bear send for the man who has had a vision giving him arrow wound power. His face painted with streaks of yellow and white, as his vision directed, this "doctor" comes to the door of the sick man's te-pee, singing the song he dreamed. He paints the face of the patient and ties an eagle plume to his hair. He bids all the young men help in singing his powerful song, while he dances and strikes the ground with a buffalo tail. Then he and the patient bathe in the river. It was a clean wound and it heals.[28]

In the same geographical region, a few select men of the great Oglala Dakota tribe belonged to the secret Sacred Bow Society. The four holy bows that belonged to the group were never used for hunt-ing or warfare. Each bow was about four and a half feet long, and all four were alike except for the kind of wood used in their construction. "The bow was double-curved and unstrung," reported Helen H. Blish. "Rattlesnake skins wrapped the wood, and strips of sinew were strung along it, bound firmly at the center of the two curves and at the handle at the center of the bow." Eagle plumes and medicine bags also deco-rated the instrument, as did a striking feather banner that hung from one end. A rattlesnake skin was suspended from the banner near the bow, "and from the lower tip of the banner hung two eagle tail feath-ers, attached to it by ribbons of bear gut." During ceremonies the bow was carried in the left hand of a member of the Sacred Bow Society, but at all other times it was carried in the crook of the left arm.

> At no time was it allowed to touch the ground, for it was sacred; and it was kept away from women. When out for ceremonial performances, it had to be laid upon sage. . . . On other occa-sions it was kept in a strip of buffalo hide painted red, into which it must be placed ceremonially. Always before use it was passed through the smoke of burning sweet-grass to purify it.[29]

The members of the Sacred Bow Society concerned themselves mainly with preparing for war. They met high standards of strength

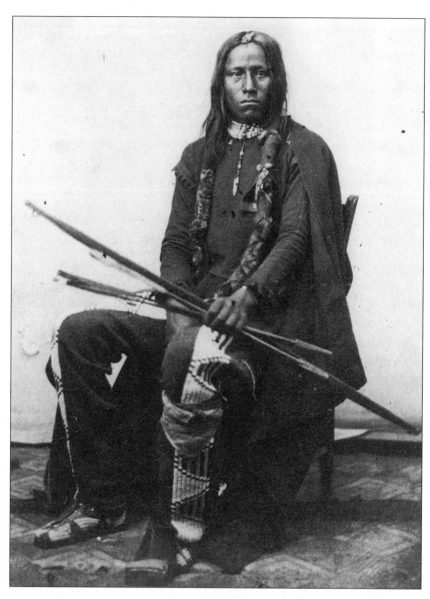

Unidentified Sioux chief, ca. 1868–69. Note the length of the arrow points. (Photo by Jackson Bros.; courtesy Museum of New Mexico, #139528)

and courage, were regarded with special esteem, and were actually the philosophers of the tribe. The symbolism of the sacred bow was so strong that it might have been considered to be the emblem of a healing society. Oddly, the bows were essentially "war medicine."

The Paiutes of southeastern Utah believed that when the world was young three great monsters roamed the earth destroying corn crops, driving off game, and killing human beings. The Paiutes were too weak and unskilled in warfare to challenge the monsters or protect themselves against the evil these beasts caused. At long last, however, the Paiute god Shinob came to their rescue. Grabbing a rainbow, he molded it into a mighty bow and uprooted full-grown trees from the earth as his arrows. For tips, he used lightning. Armed with these weapons, Shinob defeated the monsters and brought peace to the world.[30]

In the Pacific Northwest, some arrow shamans used "medicine arrows" as part of healing ceremonies. The Klamath Lake and Modoc Indians of southwestern Oregon designated special arrows to be used only for curing or treating patients. During a healing ceremony, the arrows, each two to three feet long and made of any of a number of woods, were believed to receive a spirit through the healer. The healer stuck them into the ground, one on each side of the patient, who lay prone. These arrows kept the person's soul intact and scared away the disease or pinned it down and killed it. If the arrows were handled in the correct manner, the patient would recover within a short time, but pulling them up before the sick person was entirely well would either kill the patient or make him as sick as he was previously. "Any kind of songs can be sung to them [the arrows] while they stand there for days and days,"[31] reported one non-Indian observer of the ceremonies. Often the medicine people sang songs about spiders, lightning, clouds, or the wind, believing that the medicine arrows appreciated these topics.

In these two tribes another, different arrow sometimes complemented the first type, depending on whether the healer thought it was necessary. The second arrow improved the medical power of the healer by calling up animal spirits who would help the shaman become a stronger doctor. The increased ability to heal came during a dance that lasted five days and five nights. During this time, the special arrow caught the patient's disease. The healer then took it to a deep pit where it was destroyed. Symbolically, of course, the ailment was also then defeated.

The mighty Cheyenne derive their life and power from four medicine arrows—red, white, yellow, and black—that occupy the center of

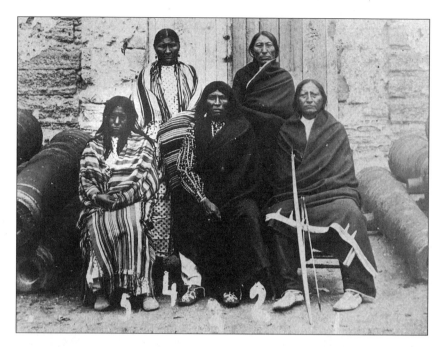

Sioux and Cheyenne prisoners at Fort San Marcos, ca. 1875–78. Note bow and arrow in front of Chief Minimac. (Courtesy St. Augustine Historical Society, #SAH2-3541)

a creation myth along with a Cheyenne culture hero named Sweet Medicine. Sweet Medicine's mother carried this beautiful boy in her womb for four years. Not long after giving birth she and her husband died, and Sweet Medicine's grandmother took him in and raised him. As a young man he traveled to a sacred mountain called Bear Butte, near the Black Hills. When the youth neared the mountain, a door opened and he went inside. He stayed for four years after having been told he was to become the prophet of the Cheyenne. During these years Sweet Medicine learned the sacred Cheyenne ceremonies, songs, magic, and prophecies, and he received a bundle containing four medicine arrows. At the end of his time in the mountain he took all of his knowledge and the arrows back to his people.

When Sweet Medicine arrived at the Cheyenne camp, he found his tribe weak from hunger, for a famine had swept the countryside. Sweet Medicine immediately ordered that a tepee be erected in the center of the camp. He gathered the elders and the holy people inside the enclosure and instructed them in the mysteries he had learned inside the mountain. Two of the medicine arrows, he said, were "Buffalo Arrows" because they represented power over these creatures and other animals. They had to be used very cautiously, preferably only when the tribe was desperate for food. Then, instructed Sweet Medicine, they should search for a herd of buffalo and point the two arrows at them until the animals became confused and ran around in circles. In this condition they would be easy to kill. "Buffalo killed with the aid of the Buffalo Arrows were butchered in a prescribed way," reported Harold Ottaway. "Everything was taken except the head with the horns still on, and this must remain attached to the backbone and the tail."[32]

The other two arrows were called "Man Arrows" and were said to bring victory in battle. Before attacking, Cheyenne warriors held ceremonies in which these two arrows played a prominent role. At the conclusion of the ritual, the Arrow Keeper, who held an exalted and coveted position in the tribe, pointed the two arrows in the direction of the enemy. The enemy soldiers were blinded by the arrows' power, and thus their effectiveness in battle was greatly diminished.

Collectively, these medicine arrows are called "Mahuts," after the name of the Cheyenne creator, Maheo. Maheo presented the arrows to Sweet Medicine while he was inside the mountain, and through him to all the Cheyenne, with the understanding that they bound the Indians to the All Father. In turn, the All Father originally gave life to the Plains Indians through the sacred arrows. Without them, it is understood, there can be no Cheyenne tribe and no Cheyenne people in any supernatural sense. These arrows were also looked upon as the supreme symbols and sources of Cheyenne male power. Out of respect, the Mahuts were housed in a particular tepee and guarded by a society of Cheyenne men who were known as Arrow Keepers.

In the summer of 1830 the sacred arrows led the tribe in warfare against the Pawnee. Trouble had been developing for years between the two neighboring tribes, and bloody battles had been fought. This time, however, unequivocal victory for the Cheyenne was practically guaranteed because the arrows, carried by White Thunder's wife on her back, were leading the group into Pawnee territory. At that time White Thunder was the Arrow Keeper, and his wife symbolized the wife of Sweet Medicine, the first arrow bearer. The faces and hands of both were covered with red paint, in obedience to the instructions given by Maheo to Sweet Medicine and his woman inside the Holy Mountain.[33]

The hostile encounter with the Pawnee occurred suddenly and without warning, however, and White Thunder had no time to conduct the ceremonies that would have ensured a Cheyenne victory. Had time been on their side, he would have laid the medicine arrows on a bed of white sage, he would have elevated them slowly until their points were aimed at the hearts and heads of the enemy, he would have danced and chanted and thrust the arrows into the air, the warriors would have shouted each time White Thunder performed a certain ceremonial exercise, and White Thunder would have aimed the arrows at the earth. But the surprise confrontation prevented these ceremonies from taking place. So, without the power of the ritual behind him, White Thunder quickly fastened the Mahuts to the lance of Bull, the priest-warrior who would carry them into battle against the Pawnee.

Among the Pawnee, it is said, lived an old and sick man, ready to die. He willingly sat in the front of the Pawnee line of warriors, singing a death song, with his bows and arrows nearby. Bull ignored warnings not to go near the old man. Instead, he attempted to touch the ailing Pawnee, but he was fooled. The old man moved the trunk of his body, grabbed Bull's extended lance, and pulled it from his hand. Pawnee warriors, recognizing the arrow bundle and knowing its value to the Cheyenne, quickly took it from the man's hands and rode off with it. Proudly, they handed their chief the sacred trophy. The Pawnee leader gleefully fastened it to his lance and rode back toward the Cheyenne with the intention of embarrassing them. He succeeded. Totally demoralized, the Cheyenne retreated.

In time the Cheyenne called a new council, who decided to consecrate four new arrows, resembling exactly those given to the Cheyenne by Maheo and subsequently captured by the Pawnee. Before the new arrows were carved, however, peaceable efforts were made to acquire the original icons from the Pawnee. After much pleading and begging by the Cheyenne, the Pawnee chief finally agreed to give back one of the arrows. Some time later, perhaps in 1837, the Brule Sioux attacked a Pawnee village and recovered another of the sacred arrows for their Cheyenne allies. For years afterward, all efforts by the Cheyenne to obtain the two remaining sacred arrows failed. As late as 1866 the Cheyenne promised to make peace with the Pawnees and to give

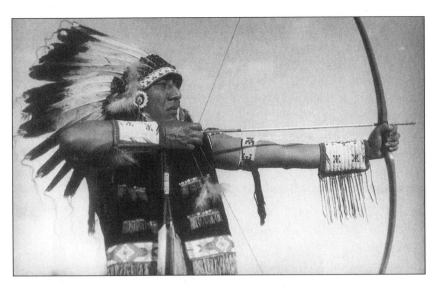

Pawnee Chief Lone Bear, ca. 1935. (Photo by Harold Kellogg; courtesy Museum of New Mexico, #77515)

them a hundred fine horses plus other gifts if the captured arrows were returned. The offer was refused. From that time until May 1931, when General Hugh Scott said that the arrows were still in Pawnee hands, all efforts at acquiring the original two arrows were unsuccessful. Nonetheless, the two old and two new arrows are venerated by the Cheyenne and are considered sacred.

In the Cheyenne way, regardless of whether the arrows are old or new, oaths taken on them are inviolate. Assurances given in the presence of the arrows must be kept; promises made must be honored; pledges must be respected. To do otherwise, according to the people, is to bring down the wrath of Maheo. That is what happened to brevet Major General George Custer. The Cheyenne said that Custer lied to them about many things, including the intentions of the military, as he smoked with Stone Forehead, then the Arrow Keeper, beneath the sacred arrows themselves in 1869. Not long afterward, Custer lay dead in the dust and heat of the Little Bighorn battlefield and the Cheyenne and Sioux rode away victorious.[34]

There is another version of the story of the Pawnees' theft of the sacred arrows, written in 1903. The circumstances of battle between the Cheyenne and the Pawnee are similar in this tale, including the events up to the time when the old Pawnee man grabbed the lance from the Cheyenne warrior. In this tale, however, the four sacred arrows were wrapped in a coyote hide—not a major difference. But the Pawnee chief is said to have kept only two arrows, the black one and the red. The yellow and white arrows were given to another Pawnee warrior. For years afterward the Cheyenne invited the Pawnee to visit them and asked them to bring the arrows. When the old Pawnee chief obliged and paid calls, however, he carried only one arrow—the red one. The other, the black one, he left behind because he believed it had much more meaning than the others.

During one of his visits, the aging leader incautiously placed the red arrow on the ground and a Cheyenne man leaped up from the rear of the circle, picked up the red arrow, and ran off with it. Sometime afterward, the Cheyenne captured the white and yellow arrows, but according to this rendition, the black arrow was never returned.[35]

A third version contains a bit more information about the sick old man. His ailment, it seems, involved sores that the medicine man was unable to cure. The sores, which covered the old man's body, were months old and so severe that they prevented him from standing. He decided it would be better for all if he died in battle, so when the Cheyenne approached, the man asked his brothers and uncles to place him in front of the line of warriors. Agreeing, his male relatives carried him, sitting on a robe, to a spot where he would be exposed to the Cheyenne arrows. They spread a strong bow and many arrows in front of the old man so that he could defend himself if he chose.

A Cheyenne warrior carrying a lance painted with white clay that had a small coyote hide–covered bundle attached charged at the sick man. When the Cheyenne was close enough, the Pawnee elder reached up and yanked the spear from his hand. He then stuck it in the ground until the Pawnee chief, Big Eagle, pulled it out and handed it to one of his warriors to take back to the camp.

After the battle, Big Eagle examined the spear and found that it consisted of a "long wooden shaft, wrapped with strips of otter hide, with an iron head at one end . . . close to the head and wrapped about the shaft was a bundle of arrows in a coyote hide."[36] As the chief was looking at the booty, one of the old man's kin came in and demanded the spear. The chief, a generous leader, turned the spear and one arrow over to the relative. Later, after a ceremony, the coyote hide and three arrows were made part of a Pawnee sacred medicine bundle. Two years later the Cheyenne attacked again, this time entering the village and finding the old man still alive. They killed him then and took back the one arrow that had been given to his relative.

The Cheyenne made many more attempts to regain their arrows. All failed, and, according to the legend, the Pawnee still have at least two of the sacred Cheyenne arrows.

Within many Native American cultures, the power of arrows— actual or symbolic—can define a people. Often, the arrows a warrior carried into battle in his quiver were held to be a sacred gift from the Creator. The arrows protected the tribe; they guided through example; they healed through their medicine; and they connected Indian souls to an all-encompassing Indian spirit. It is no wonder that Native Americans used arrows so expertly to defend their beliefs. After all, so many facets of tribal life were associated with arrows, especially those that represented the Creator. In that sense, nothing in modern weaponry even comes close.

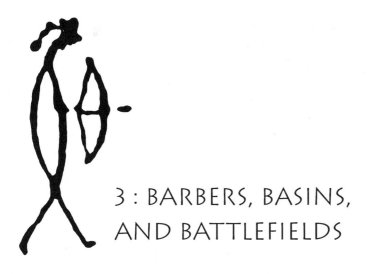

3 : BARBERS, BASINS, AND BATTLEFIELDS

Fortunately for everyone, Indians no longer ride into battle carrying arrows that kill. Natives and soldiers no longer need traditional healers and military physicians to treat the wounds of the Indian wars. This is not to say that America's armed forces no longer have a role to play in United States history. Young fliers, soldiers, sailors, and marines are still dedicated to preserving democracy in the world. The men and women of the United States armed forces cut a proud swath across the pages of history as they risk their lives, sometimes in very unpopular wars. And within their ranks are brave physicians, the linear descendants of a group of medical men whose devotion to helping and healing brought them to the frontier West and Southwest.

But the military surgeons assigned to Indian country in the 1800s were themselves only the latest in a long line of healers who began their work as barbers centuries earlier in Europe. The transition from barber to physician came about slowly. The payment of a certain tax entitled forward-looking individuals to establish and operate businesses offering a new concept: personal bodily cleanliness. Before the Middle Ages, frequent bathing was unpopular, to say the least, but events took a turn for the better, and bathing in a variety of ways became fashionable—and communal. Sweat baths, water and herb baths, and mineral water baths became the mode.

A new profession arose to meet the demand for bathhouses. The duties of the owner-bathman in the public bathing houses ranged from operating the facility, to heating the water, to hair-cutting and shaving, to supervising his staff of bathhouse employees. Their low social status prevented the latter from enrolling in an organized guild, as their employers, the bathhouse owners, did, and management positions were beyond them. They could, however, legitimately provide other services, including shaving patrons, treating minor wounds, reducing fractures, and bloodletting. These workers, variously called barbers or wound surgeons or barber-surgeons, eventually formed their own guild and coexisted cooperatively with the organized groups of businessmen who had formerly been their employers.

Like modern physicians, the licensed physicians practicing in the 1600s preferred to locate in metropolitan areas. A city of ten thousand inhabitants might have two or three doctors providing health care to its residents. Citizens of rural areas, however, neither the most appealing nor the most profitable sites for newly graduated physicians, continued to rely on barber-surgeons for health care. In any case, the more learned doctors of that time were interested only in diagnosing, not in healing, possibly because cures were so rare. If a physician's patients died, his reputation might suffer, so it is easy to see why he might avoid taking any on in the first place. Thus, regardless of the place, the treatment of certain ailments by cupping (an ancient way of bloodletting accomplished by applying drinking glasses to the body to draw blood to the surface), for example, was usually turned over to barber-surgeons.[1]

A 1658 engraving of a barber-surgeon's shop in a Dutch city depicts the medical equipment then available to combat illness.[2] Two shaving basins, a chain of extracted teeth with a large artificial tooth in the middle, and a live bird in a cage complement benches and tables covered with cloths.

Another illustration, a painting, shows a village doctor's shop circa 1640, with unusual decor: stuffed fishes and crocodiles, skulls, dead armadillos, and a live owl flying around the room. Also depicted in this work of art are two apprentices. One is preparing ointments while six individuals watch the pain-contorted face of a patient undergoing a minor head operation.

A century and a half later, conditions had improved. A 1790 engraving portrays an upper-class urban barbershop. Cleanliness is obvious. The tables are covered with white cloths, as are the customers themselves. Surgical instruments and dental forceps hang neatly on the walls beside enema syringes, pewter measuring vessels, and apothecaries' containers. The barber-surgeon has treated a man with his arm in a sling and is now performing a dental procedure. On one table are a lamp, a bandage, a basin, a hairbrush, and a mirror.

During medieval military campaigns, barber-surgeons who volunteered for duty became known as field barbers. They treated sick or wounded soldiers with state-of-the-art remedies: bloodletting, enemas, cupping, emetics, purgatives, cauterization, and amputations. Special forceps had been designed to probe for bullets. Not until the end of the eighteenth century was an effort made in Europe to separate barber-surgeons on the battlefield from formally educated physicians also serving in the military. By the nineteenth century, the barber-surgeons had disappeared completely from most modern armies, with the exception of the Russian army. Across the Atlantic, soldiers in the expanding American armies were treated by doctors of the newly created medical corps. Nonmilitary physicians as well were becoming prominent, some as doctor-statesmen and advisers to presidents.

Dr. Benjamin Rush, a noted Philadelphia physician in the early 1800s, played an essential part in preparing members of the Lewis and Clark expedition for their hazardous journey into the northern West, home to many unpredictable Indian tribes. At the request of President Thomas Jefferson, Dr. Rush developed a list of questions about Indians that Captain Meriwether Lewis was to personally answer at the end of the group's journey up the Missouri River.[3] Rush's inquiries, several of which relate to bilious fevers and diseases, were surprisingly naïve, given the uncertainty of what lay ahead for the explorers. Apparently no thought was given to potential hostility from the Indian groups along the way, nor were encounters with the native people even considered three weeks later when another list prepared by Dr. Rush was presented to Captain Lewis.[4] Entitled "Dr. Rush to Capt. Lewis, for preserving his health, June 11, 1803," the list of eleven suggestions includes no measures to be taken should the party confront unfriendly natives and be wounded by their arrows. Instead, Lewis was advised to rest, ingest purging pills, eat sparingly, wear flannel, drink molasses or sugar water, wash his feet every morning in cold water, lie down for two hours after a long march, and wear low-heeled shoes. Fortunately, most of the Indians along the route were friendly and, in part thanks to the presence of Sacajawea, gave the party a wide berth.

Members of the medical profession were present at well-known episodes in the history of the West. The three army surgeons present at the Little Big Horn on the fateful days of June 25 and 26, 1876, squarely faced their destiny. One of them, Dr. George Edwin Lord, was himself ill with trail colic and had difficulty keeping up with General Custer.[5] Despite his ailment, and Custer's suggestion that he remain in the rear, Lord rode with the general and lost his life. Dr. James M. DeWolf had been wounded at the Civil War battle of Bull Run and was receiving a pension for his injuries. Bored, he reenlisted and was assigned to the Seventh Cavalry. On June 25, Dr. DeWolf was riding with Major Marcus Reno and became separated from him. It was a fatal mistake. A third physician with the ill-fated troop, Dr. Henry Renaldo Porter, later found DeWolf's body and buried him. Porter himself was trapped on a hilltop with Reno, but in the midst of the melee he courageously established a hospital in the center of a circle of mules and horses. In a subsequent letter to his parents, Porter related that

> the wounded were brought faster than I could attend them. Men and animals were killed and wounded all around me, and the horses fell over on my wounded men. . . . One man who volunteered [to help the doctor] was shot through the leg, both knees crushed and the fleshy parts lacerated so that I had to amputate the leg below the knee.[6]

It is not known how many of the fatalities on both sides of this infamous battle were caused by guns, lances, or arrows. However, history records that a Sioux chief named Gall and his warriors stayed at the rear of the action and crawled close to L Troop. There they

> picked the soldiers off one by one, mostly with bows and arrows. A warrior thus armed could hug the ground and shoot without sound or smoke to reveal his position, and without show-

ing himself at all. He would fire up into the air, the arrow arching high on its trajectory and falling to strike a soldier silently in the back. . . . Many . . . died that way, and in death lay face down, an arrow rigid and upright in his back.[7]

Although the surgical equipment necessary for doctors to perform their tasks on the battlefield varied considerably from the equipment used by physicians in private practice, military physicians all had one thing in common: a shaving basin. Along with this indispensable vessel company surgeons often carried the following:

> a blood-letting set consisting of a case with a scarification knife and six extra blades, one sponge, a scarlet bandage, six other bandages, a bag with straight and curved scissors, a pair of plaster shears, a sponge forceps, a straight grooved probe, a chest probe, a bistouri, one spatula and one spoon, a tourniquet with accompanying accessories, a small box with needles and ligatures, bandage material, two cardboard boxes with drugs, three bottles with liquid drugs.

On the other hand, the field chest of a regimental surgeon contained

> several razors, two bistouries, several lancets for blood-letting and the opening of abscesses, two scissors for bandages and incisions, a clasp knife, a bone saw, forceps, two bullet drawers (with which to bore into and withdraw lead bullets), all sorts of probes, suture needles with accessories, two syringes with long cannulas, a complete trepan, enema syringes, a sponge, and a mortar.

In addition, for compresses the physician had "a small cask filled with linen fibres, a cask of old linen cloths and shirts, four dozen napkins, all kinds of prepared bandages, several dozen crutches, sticks, and cots."[8]

Army ambulances made their first appearance in 1859; before that, mule-drawn wagons were used to transport the wounded—and only 180 wagons were in service in 1847. Other shortcomings on the new frontier included a complete lack of shelters or hospital tents and very few pieces of equipment or medical supplies other than what military physicians carried in their bags. After the Civil War, however, the situation improved. The medical corps became fairly well organized, and although medicines and implements were still scarce, particularly on the frontier, little by little army surgeons became able to provide reasonable clinical care, among their other, more mundane duties—and other duties there were.

Fort Davis was located near Limpia Creek in the Davis Mountains of west Texas. The fort had been abandoned during most of the Civil War but was reactivated as a military outpost in 1867 by a detachment of the new black Ninth Cavalry. One year later, on December 18, 1868, thirty-year-old Assistant Surgeon Daniel Weisel reported to Fort Davis for duty.[9] As he was the only surgeon in attendance, Weisel's tasks were varied, and they were not always medical in nature. He was responsible for frequent inspections of all physical properties and living areas, the water supply, and cooking equipment.

> He was to detect all sources of sickness and poor sanitation, and to try to convince a frequently preoccupied post command of the need for correction in problem areas . . . he was responsible for the post cemetery, for making regular sick calls, supervising the pharmacy, treating patients, examining recruits,

and for overseeing the performance of related personnel such as cooks, matrons, and nurses. The doctor's obligations also extended to keeping records, making daily reports, and dealing with amazing volumes of paperwork, especially so considering the uncomplicated, isolated, and remote nature of the outpost. He was the post treasurer and bakery supervisor.

One of Dr. Weisel's missions was to stay ahead of the unsanitary conditions at Fort Davis. Deplorable sanitation practices existed there—and in most military facilities—due primarily to the men's lack of knowledge regarding hygienic measures. Weisel reported that "filthy" conditions prevailed in the fort's kitchens, water was in short supply, and garbage and trash were thrown everywhere. Personal cleanliness among the troops was also lacking, exacerbated by the inconvenience of hauling water from Limpia Creek. In time the creek, the sole source of water for the troops, became contaminated by drainage from the stables.

The dirt-floor barracks at the fort were "very untidy, dirty, and disorderly." The guardhouse was overcrowded and poorly ventilated. In report after report, Dr. Weisel recommended disinfection and forcing the prisoners to bathe.

Most of the soldiers, whether incarcerated or not, suffered from several ailments, but Weisel's principal concern was the widespread scurvy, a disease caused by a deficiency of ascorbic acid (vitamin C). Scurvy occurs when fresh fruit and vegetables are lacking from the diet, a common situation in military encampments. The first sign of scurvy is bleeding gums. Although this may not seem terribly serious, if the condition is not corrected, previously healed wounds open and bleed, anemia occurs, and extreme weakness results. If left untreated, scurvy leads to death. Troops with a malady such as scurvy cannot be expected to mount their horses, load their weapons, and fight the good fight against a strong and skillful enemy.

In his early months as post surgeon, the doctor urged the troops to eat the watercress, a natural source of vitamin C, growing in nearby Limpia Creek, and he prevailed on the post adjutant to establish post and hospital gardens. A temporary hospital had been partly constructed but was not finished. Patients were admitted, but their medical problems worsened each time rains drenched the building and snows covered it with drifts. The hospital's windows couldn't be closed and were covered only with sheets. The roof leaked, and the walls were crumbling.

Many patients had been admitted to this military hospital with illnesses directly derived from their poor dietary habits and disgusting living conditions. Diarrhea was a great problem, as were fevers, respiratory diseases, syphilis, and the ever-present scurvy. Contusions, burns, dislocations, and fractures were common. During the entire period of Weisel's tenure, from 1868 through 1872, only twelve patients with gunshot wounds were hospitalized.[10] No mention was made of any soldiers who had been wounded by arrows.

The physical conditions at Arizona's first Fort Bowie were no better at the time. Describing the outpost in 1863, one military man wrote to another:

> The quarters, if it is not an abuse of language to call them such, have been constructed without system, regard to health, de-

fense or convenience. Those occupied by the men are mere hovels, mostly excavations in the side hill, damp, illy ventilated, and covered with decomposed granite taken from the excavation, through which the rain passes very much as it would through a sieve.[11]

Documents show that until 1868, Fort Bowie was a ramshackle collection of stone-and-adobe huts thrown across a southern Arizona hillside. The threat posed to the area by the fearsome Chiricahua Apaches, some of whom at that time still used bows and arrows in warfare, became so serious, however, that a new, larger facility was constructed on a plateau southeast of the first fort. Robert Utley described it: "Substantial barracks, a row of houses for officers, corrals and storehouses, a post trader's store, and a commodious hospital soon occupied the four sides of the sloping parade ground. In subsequent years, more buildings were added."[12]

Twenty years later, at Fort Sill, Oklahoma, the general situation regarding sanitation was much the same. The enlisted men's barracks reeked from the aroma of urine steadily crystallizing in the stone outhouses behind the living quarters. Kitchen refuse was emptied into one of many drains on the post. From time to time, a ditch running behind the soldiers' barracks and not too far from the latrines became clogged with grease, meat scraps, and other food wastes. Swarms of flies and mosquitoes brought illness to all the post personnel, but especially the enlisted men. It is not unreasonable to conclude that the military surgeons, assistant surgeons, and acting assistant surgeons assigned to Fort Sill might have wished for something as "simple" to treat as arrow wounds. As it was, malaria was rampant, followed closely by diphtheria and typhoid. When at last the order came to empty and clean the gullies crisscrossing the military reserve, an estimated 135 tons of garbage, trash, and manure was removed![13]

When a soldier stationed at a military facility became ill or was wounded, he was hospitalized in the post hospital. While the physical conditions there were not much dissimilar to those of his living quarters, he might at least escape temporarily from the putrid smells that swirled around inside his barracks—that is, unless the stench of a fellow soldier's decaying flesh, infected from an arrow wound or two, greeted him as he entered the medical ward and took his place among the long row of cots.

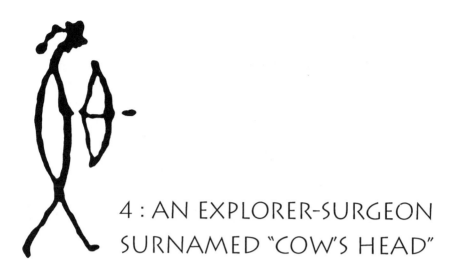

4 : AN EXPLORER-SURGEON
SURNAMED "COW'S HEAD"

The first treatment of arrow wounds by non-Indians in the American West or Southwest probably occurred sometime between June and December 1535, not far from the Rio Grande. In what is now either far west Texas or northern Mexico, a bedraggled, emaciated, and exhausted Spaniard with an unusual name collapsed to the ground, rested, and then started to write in his journal:

Here they brought a man to me and said that a long time ago he had been wounded with an arrow through the right shoulder, and the arrowhead was lodged over the heart. He said that it gave him much pain and for that reason he was always sick. I touched him, felt the arrowhead, and saw that it traversed the cartilage. With a knife I had, I opened his chest to that spot and saw that the point was crosswise and was very difficult to remove. I continued to cut, inserted the point of the knife, and with great difficulty I finally extracted it. It was very long. With a deer bone, using my knowledge of surgery, I took two stitches, following which he bled profusely all over me. With hair from a skin [animal] I staunched the flow of blood. When I had removed the arrowhead they asked me for it and I gave it to them. The entire village came to see it and they sent it into the back country so that all those who were there might view it. Because of this operation they had many dances and festivities, as was their custom. On another day, I cut the Indian's two stitches and he was well. The wound I had made was no more apparent than a crease in the palm of the hand. He said he felt neither pain nor any discomfort. And this cure gave us among them and throughout the land control of all that they considered valuable or cherished.[1]

This man, Alvar Núñez Cabeza de Vaca, was not a doctor; he was an explorer whom misfortune had thrust several years previously into a region that Spain would later claim as its northernmost outpost. Fortunately for Cabeza de Vaca (in Spanish, *cabeza* means "head" and *vaca* means "cow"), his untrained surgical skill was equal to the task of curing the natives of their afflictions in the new country. Had it not been, he probably would not have lived long enough to record the description quoted above in his diary.

The strange surname dates back to the thirteenth century and Spain's struggles against the Moors. Sancho, a Spanish king and military commander, found a mountain pass under tight Moorish control. He was about to order his troops to retreat when a shepherd named Martín Alhaja appeared and told him of an unguarded pass. He offered to show it to the king and promised he would mark it with a cow's skull. The Spanish army successfully crossed the pass, caught the Moor invaders off guard, and defeated them. As a reward, the king conferred a title on the shepherd and his descendants for all time—Cabeza de Vaca.[2]

Alvar Núñez Cabeza de Vaca was born in Jerez de la Frontera, Spain, sometime around 1490 to civic-minded parents. His father, Francisco de Vera, was an alderman, and his mother was Teresa Cabeza de Vaca. His paternal grandfather was Pedro de Vera Mendoza, the conqueror of the Canary Islands. The young Cabeza de Vaca entered military service and showed his valor in 1512 at the battle of Ravenna. After the battle he was promoted to lieutenant, and he returned to Seville in 1513. On February 15, 1527, he was appointed royal treasurer of the Narváez expedition to Florida, "one of the most disastrous enterprises in the annals of Spanish history."[3]

Cabeza de Vaca's *entrada* into the mysterious and mostly unexplored West is the stuff of legend. After leaving Florida the explorers

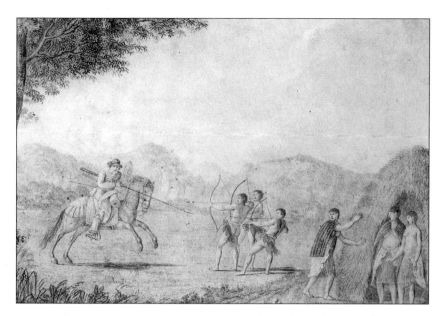

Pencil drawing of confrontation between a Spaniard and Native Americans. Sketch by Suría, member of the 1791 Malaspina Expedition. (Courtesy Museum of New Mexico, #70644)

were shipwrecked off the Texas coast, probably on Galveston Island or just west of it on Follet's Island, in 1528. Cabeza de Vaca and about 250 initial survivors were soon spotted by Indians armed with bows and arrows. When one of the explorers set out to survey the land, he was

> pursued by three Indians with bows and arrows. They were calling out to him and he was trying to speak to them through sign language. . . . He got to where we were and the Indians stayed back a bit, seated on the same shore. Half an hour later, another one hundred Indian bowmen appeared. We were so scared. . . . As best we could we tried to reassure them and ourselves, and gave them beads and little bells. Each of them gave me an arrow, which is a sign of friendship.[4]

Cabeza de Vaca and his ever-diminishing number of crewmen lived as "prisoners" among the Indians of Texas and the Southwest for six years. It was an unusual arrangement. The Spaniards were not captives in the true sense of the word, and the Indians were usually not hostile toward them. Both groups suffered from the extremely harsh environmental conditions and had to struggle side by side in order to survive that first harsh winter after the shipwreck. When the Spaniards became so hungry that they engaged in cannibalism, the natives were appalled. Paradoxically, however, the newcomers' desperate actions probably caused the Indians to regard them with respect—or fear—and changed the distribution of power toward a more equitable balance.

When spring arrived, Cabeza de Vaca was asked by the Indians to minister to those in the tribe who were ill. Noted the Spaniard,

> They wished to make us physicians without examination or inquiring for diplomas. They cure by blowing upon the sick, and with that breath and the imposing of hands they cast out infirmity. They ordered that we also should do this, and be of use to them in some way. We laughed at what they did, telling them it was folly, that we knew not how to heal. In consequence, they withheld food from us until we should practice what they required. . . . At last, finding ourselves in great want we were constrained to obey.[5]

Hunger once again dictated the Europeans' course of action.

Ever inventive, and undoubtedly scared out of his wits, Cabeza de Vaca chanted the Paternoster and the Ave Maria as he breathed on the native patients and blessed them with the sign of the cross. Miraculously, the natives' major complaints—headaches—disappeared and their diarrhea ceased. Cabeza de Vaca also successfully cauterized open, oozing sores or wounds with burning wood, all to the accompaniment of prayers in Spanish, always begging God to help him escape his predicament.

In September 1534 the heavenly petitions were answered, and he and Alonzo de Castillo, Andrés Dorantes, and their slave, Estevanico—the last of the shipwreck survivors—fled their captors. Along the way south and west they were met by scores of friendly Indians who passed them on from tribe to tribe. As long as the Spaniards could heal the natives, they were safe. One entry in Cabeza de Vaca's journal records a successful healing ceremony.

> Many Indians gathered . . . bringing five sick persons who were crippled and in a very poor condition, looking for Castillo to heal them. Each one of the sick persons offered his bow and arrows, which he accepted. At sunset he made the sign of the

cross on them and commended them to God our Lord, and we all asked God as best we could, to restore their health. . . . And God was so merciful that the following morning they all awakened well and healthy. They went away as strong as if they had never been sick. This caused great astonishment among them and caused us to thank our Lord.[6]

At long last the wanderers encountered a group of Spaniards on horseback in northern Mexico near the Gulf of California. After they managed to convince the riders that they were the lost explorers, the ragtag adventurers were guided to Mexico City. They arrived there on July 25, 1536, having survived an incredible eight-year journey that had no rival at the time in terms of drama.

One of the more remarkable aspects of the situation was that Cabeza de Vaca was considered a healer by the natives with whom he had contact. Fortunately, his description of what surely was the first surgical procedure performed by a non-Indian in the American Southwest remains for scholars to examine. But possibly even more significant than the existence of the historical record is the actual result of Cabeza de Vaca's surgery. According to Jesse Thompson, Cabeza de Vaca's skill with a knife and subsequent reputation as a physician or medicine man among Indian tribes "gave him control over the Indians and was responsible for his eventual safe return to civilization."[7]

Too bad Thompson quoted nothing from Cabeza de Vaca's journal about the type of arrowhead he removed from the Indian patient's chest. It would have been an interesting exercise to compare that tip with those that have been classified, described, and illustrated in books and journal articles in the intervening centuries. We already know a great deal about atlatls and the variety of arrowheads used by the indigenous peoples of North and South America, but Cabeza de Vaca's description would make an interesting addition.

Anthropologist Stewart Peckham of New Mexico described some of the projectiles, hand-held weapons, protective devices, and hunting tools used by indigenous peoples.[8] Beginning with the atlatl point, Peckham carefully addressed the geometry and construction of the dart and the dynamics of throwing it. The atlatl dart—the forerunner of the arrow, according to Peckham—fit snugly, attached to a foreshaft, into a spear's mainshaft. Often these dart throwers were as much as fourteen feet long, especially in the Southwest, where the Spanish influence was strong.[9] The dart tip and its shaft combined measured four to six feet in length, almost twice the size of an arrow. Peckham hypothesized that early hunters or warriors in the Southwest carried only a few mainshafts but many foreshafts and darts, possibly in animal-skin pouches.

Clarence Ellsworth, writing for the Southwest Museum in Los Angeles, described the probable evolution of the atlatl.

> The first weapons, besides teeth and claws, were no doubt clubs and stones, then pointed sticks which served as spears. Hard points were next bound to the sticks and a true spear was invented. About this time someone began to throw these spears instead of prodding with them, and in order to get a little more distance, the size was diminished. Then it was discovered that a longer arm with an extra joint could be made of another piece of wood, giving extra power and distance, and some accuracy. This implement we call a throwing stick, or *atlatl*, its Aztec name. There is no question that it was used in our Southwest before the bow made its appearance.[10]

It is difficult to reconcile Ellsworth's view with the view of those who believe bows and arrows reached the Four Corners area of the upper Southwest at the end of the Basketmaker period (about 700–900 A.D.) and spread to California much later. For obvious reasons the atlatl would have fallen into disuse as soon as bows and arrows appeared in this part of the country.

Peckham compared the smaller, lighter arrow with the earlier spear and its tip. Clearly it would be inefficient to throw an arrow like an atlatl dart, but early arrows were quite similar to darts in their construction. The mainshaft was a hollow reed, and the foreshaft was made of a harder wood such as mountain mahogany. Often a slotted wooden plug was inserted in the butt end of the mainshaft to provide a nock for the bowstring.

It is easy to envision a Native American of old, sitting in the shade of a desert willow, slowly and carefully constructing an arrow. If the warrior had a colorful personality, he probably spared no effort in decorating the arrow with the designs that popped up from his imagina-

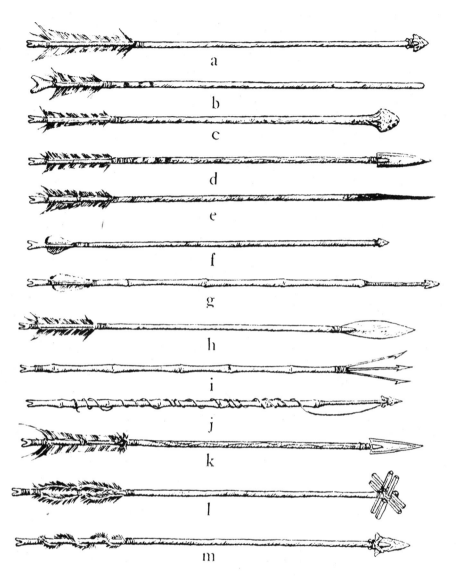

TYPES OF PRIMITIVE ARROWS: *a. Arrow with stone point. b. Child's arrow without point and with large nock. c. Knob-headed arrow—a 'bunt.' d. Typical Plains type with iron point. e. Arrow with charred point; sometimes the whole arrowshaft was scorched slightly to stiffen or produce more 'spine' in the shaft. f. Arrow with 'bird-point' of stone. g. Cane arrow with hardwood foreshaft and stone point. h. Arrow with wide iron point. i. Fish-arrow of cane, with iron points. j. Type of cane fish-arrow with removable point. k. Sioux type of arrow with iron point and grooves in shaft. l. Arrow for birds and small game, with whole feathers attached. m. Arrow with single feather spiraled around shaft and with stone point. (from Ellsworth,* Bows and Arrows *, Fig. 2).*

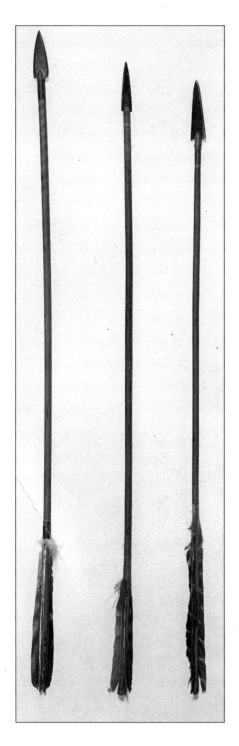

NINETEENTH-CENTURY AR-ROWS. Left: Wichita "Poison Arrow," wide flat head with sharpened edges. Center: Kiowa war arrow. Right: Sioux arrow with zigzag grooves on shaft. (Courtesy Museum of the Fur Trade Collections)

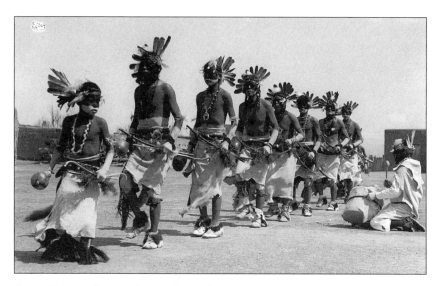

Bow and arrow dance at San Ildefonso Pueblo, New Mexico, 1932. Rituals such as this dance date back into antiquity. (Photo by Harold Kellogg; courtesy Museum of New Mexico, #77477)

tion. He would have used the colors of the desert—vegetable dyes of browns, greens, reds, yellows, and blacks—probably smeared on the shaft with his fingers or delicately stroked onto the wood with fine grasses as brushes. Feathers were always part of the arrow, taken from captured wild turkeys, prairie chickens, or, on special occasions, eagles. According to Peckham, scientific analysis has proved that the added feathers increase friction and drag. Basically, however, the technical investigators proved what the Indians already knew: arrows with feathers fly straighter.

Famed anthropologist and ethnologist Frederick W. Hodge described how feathers were used on Indian arrows. The feathers differed in the species of bird from which they came, in the kind and number used, and in their form, length, and manner of setting. Arrows might be without feathers, or they might carry two or three feathers, depending on the customs of individual tribes.[11] For example, Captain John G. Bourke, a soldier who was quite familiar with Indian tribes of the West, described the arrows made by the Apaches: "The Apaches use three hawk feathers, arranged equidistant along the shaft in the direction of the longer axis, fastened with sinew."[12] Hawk feath-

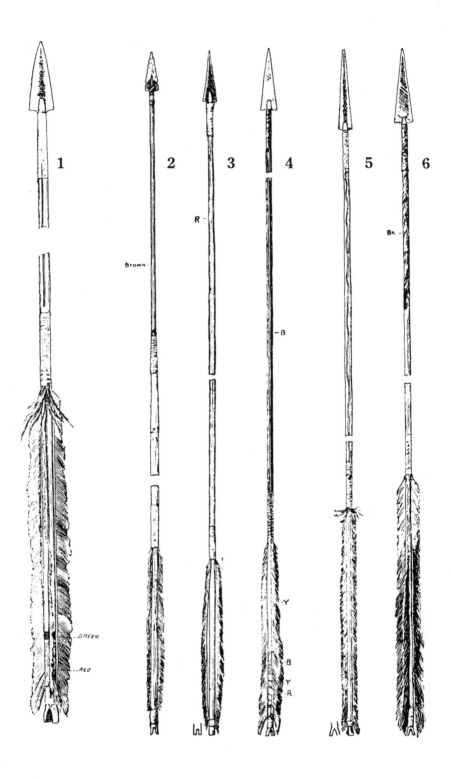

ARROWS OF APACHE TRIBES, SOUTHWESTERN UNITED STATES. FIG. 1. *The shaft is of osier, with shaft streaks nearly straight. Shaftment tapering backwards and banded with red and green paint. Nock, swallow-tail shaped. Feathers, three, seized at their ends with sinew and extending off from the shaft at the middle. The front part of the feathering is ornamented with tufts of down. The delicate blade of iron forming the head is inserted into a "saw cut" in the end of the shaft and seized with sinew. Total length, 25 1/2 inches. Cat. No. 6964, U.S.N.M. Comanche Indians of Texas. Collected by Dr. E. Palmer, U.S. Army. FIG. 2. Shaft, of reed. The shaftment is ornamented with bands of red and black. Feathers, three, seized with sinew. Notch, parallel-sided. The foreshaft of hard wood, fits into the end of the reed shaft and is seized with sinew. It is daubed with brown paint. Head, of jasper, incurved at the base and notched on the sides. It is inserted into the end of the foreshaft and fastened by a diagonal seizing of sinew and further secured by mesquite gum. Total length of shaft, 37 1/2 inches. Cat. No. 5519, U.S.N.M. Apache Indians, of Arizona. Collected by Dr. Edward Palmer. FIG. 3. SHAFT, of rhus, painted red. Feathers, three, seized with sinew, standing off from the shaftment. The nock is cylindrical and the notch is rectangular. Head, of old hoop iron, inserted in a notch in the end of the shaft and seized with sinew. This specimen is very roughly made. The total length of the shaft is 25 inches. Cat. No. 25512, U.S.N.M. Apache Indians. Collected by Dr. J. B. White, U.S. Army. FIG. 4. SHAFT, of hard wood. Iron head let in at the end of the shaft. Feathers, three, seized with sinew. Shaft painted blue. Shaftment bound with yellow, blue, and red streaks. Length, shaft, 2 feet 4 inches. Cat. No. 130307, U.S.N.M. Apache Indians. Athapascan stock. Arizona. Collected by Dr. T. C. Scantling, U.S. Army. FIG. 5. Shaft, of osier. Has three shaft streaks, two nearly straight and one a wavy line. The shaftment is ornamented with bands of red and blue. Feathers, three, attached at their ends by a seizing of sinew and glued to the shaft. Near the seizing is a bunch of downy feathers, left for the purpose of ornamentation. Nock, widely spread. Notch, angular. The head is a tapering blade of iron, a portion of which, with the tang, is inserted into a "saw cut" and neatly seized with sinew. Total length, 27 inches. FIG. 6. This arrow is similar to No. 5 A, excepting a little ornamentation on the front of the shaft, total length, 24 1/2 inches. NOTE.—Both of these arrows are perfect of their kind. It is difficult to conceive how a more deadly missile could be made. Cat. No. A and B 150450, U.S.N.M. Navajo Indians. Collected by Dr. Washington Matthews, U.S. Army. (PLATE XLIII, Smithsonian Report, 1893)*

ers, however, might not have been absolutely necessary. When on the run from the army, it would have been a frivolous (and deadly) waste of time to trap or catch hawks and then remove their feathers. During war, any creature with feathers might have been a satisfactory source.

Many tribes were, and are, quite fussy about the kinds of feathers they used to help their arrows fly accurately. Eskimos, for example, lay flat two whole feathers on the inner end of the arrow, usually with the underside of the feather outward. These they attach to the soft wood of the shaft by punching holes in the latter and inserting the ends of the feathers in these holes. Among the Salishan tribes in the Northwest, reported anthropologist Otis T. Mason,

> two whole feathers are attached to the soft cedar arrowshaft by lashings of bark. All the California arrows have three half-feathers set on radially, and in some of them there is a decided spiral in the application; but around the mouth of the Colorado River and in the mountain region of Mexico, below the boundary line, the two flat feathers occur again.[13]

Dr. Saxton T. Pope, an instructor in surgery and research at the University of California Medical School, developed a strong interest in Native American bows and arrows and in 1923 published a book about them. He addressed feathering quite briefly, stating that "the speed of rotation given an arrow varies according to the size and concavity of the feathers. It is more rapid in target arrows than in heavy shafts, for heavy heads require more feather surface to turn them than do cylindrical points."[14] Might early Native Americans have had some idea of the physics of arrow feathering? This is not an idle question. The Indians were certainly well informed about the construction of bows.

Peckham believed that bows were originally less refined than the arrows, being rather crudely made of local hardwoods, although decorated, if time permitted, with painted bands of red, black, and green, or one particular solid color. Most bows used by Native Americans on the frontier were of simple construction, usually made from one piece of wood, a type known in the vernacular as a "self-bow." The best bows, according to T. N. Hamilton, are made from Osage orange.[15] But that wood isn't available everywhere, and artisans had to rely on local trees for their materials.

Shaping the bow, or "tillering" it, is very important for a good bow. And although many studies have been conducted to determine the ideal cast of a bow, its draw, and its ratio—and the proper measurements are known—Native Americans on the frontier had only to feel what was right and what was wrong about a bow. Many modern Indian men and women can still do that. Geronimo's son Robert, for example, searched the woods surrounding the Mescalero Apache Reservation

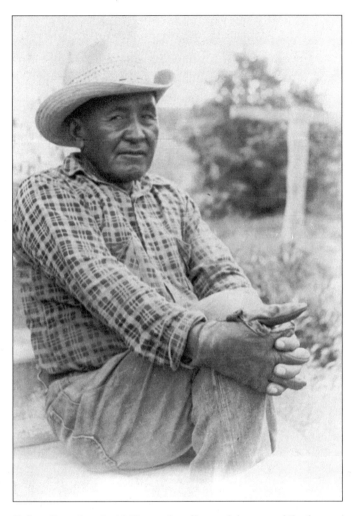

Robert Geronimo in 1948 was the only surviving son of the famous Chiricahua Apache warrior and medicine man. Geronimo crafted bows and arrows to sell to tourists visiting the reservation. (Courtesy Rev. Robert S. Ove)

in the 1950s for the perfect limb still growing on a tree. Then he tillered it, letting it grow in position until he knew it was ready. After Robert had cut the shaped limb, he finished the bow by whittling the wood with the serrated edge of a tin can lid.[16]

The bows Robert Geronimo crafted were modeled after those used when the Chiricahua Apaches were still a free people in the hills of

Arizona and New Mexico. But Robert's handiwork was never used as his forefathers' work was used—for the hunt or in battle. No, his bows (with arrows) were sold for a pittance to tourists passing through the reservation. If any still exist today, tucked away in attics, trunks, or the backs of closets, they are priceless.

Hamilton classified native bows into several categories: (1) the self-bow, which depends on the elasticity of one piece of wood for its cast; (2) the reinforced bow, essentially a self-bow with sinew or some other organic material glued to its back for added power; and (3) the composite bow, "in which horn or antler has been substituted for the wood in the belly half of the limbs and sinew [is substituted] for the back half."[17] Hamilton believed that the Apaches used a reinforced bow for hunting and warfare, although he qualified this somewhat by adding that all bows used by Apaches might not have been made by them. Bows made by the various tribes made their way around the countryside through intertribal trading and warfare. Nonetheless, he carefully described the typical Apache bow. It was "44½ inches long overall, with 43½ inches between the nocks. . . . The stave is of white oak . . . the center of the grip is 22 inches from the upper tip and measures $1\,5/32$ x $3/4$ inches. Eleven inches from the two tips the limb measures $11/32$ x $5/8$ inches; 1 inch below the upper nock the measurement is $11/16$ x $1/2$ inches, and 1 inch above the lower nock it measures $11/16$ x $17/32$ of an inch."[18]

Dr. Cyril Courville put it much more simply: "With the Apaches, the length of the bow was specifically measured, being eight times the span of the thumb to the little finger."[19] Courville also made note of the various woods for bows available to the Indians who lived and roamed along the Mexican border, which included bois d'arc, juniper, willow, cottonwood, and mesquite.

To prove his point about the power of the Apache bow, Hamilton quoted Captain John C. Bourke. In 1871 while on duty in the field, Bourke was ambushed by Apaches and shot at with arrows. Two of them hit a pine tree and penetrated to a depth of at least six inches, according to Bourke, who also believed Apache arrows could be effective at 150 yards. Hamilton disputed Bourke's claim, but Reginald and Gladys Laubin, in their *American Indian Archery*, quoted other sources as saying that "Apache arrows could pierce a man at three hundred paces."[20]

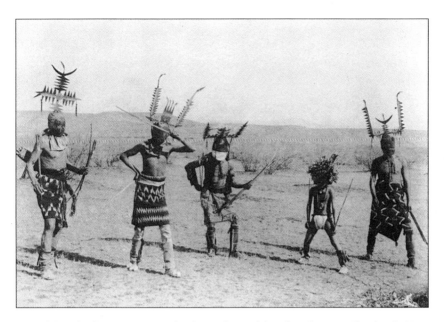

Sacred Apache dancers representing benevolent spirits often dance to dispel evil. Note bows and arrows carried by dancers at left and in center. (Courtesy Smithsonian Institution, National Museum of Natural History, National Anthropological Archives, #41-106-B)

In another document, Bourke described Apache arrows as being

composed of three distinct parts—the reed, the stem, and the barb; the last affixed to the stem, and the stem, of hard wood, inserted in the reed, and both held firmly in place by ligatures of sinew. The stem was made of a hard wood called "kk-ing" and the reed in Apache "klo-ka," meaning "arrow grass." There is a great advantage in the use of this reed, because the arrow afterwards needs no straightening, whereas the arrows made by the Zunis [a Pueblo Indian group] and others must be subjected to a special process to make them shoot true. . . . The arrow of the Apache sometimes terminates in a triangular piece of hard wood, which seems to be perfectly effective as a weapon.[21]

The Laubins quoted Bourke as saying that Apaches "seldom used the sinew-backed bow," adding, however, that all the Apache bows they themselves had seen were sinew-backed, and most were wrapped with sinew at the ends.[22] Actually, there may be no contradiction here.

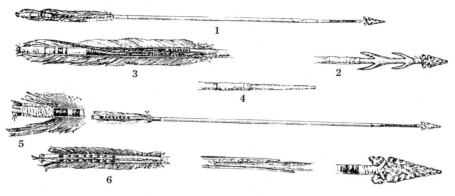

THE PARTS OF AN ARROW. The dissected arrow is shown in such fashion that the parts of a highly complex example may be understood. A COMPLETE ARROW. Foreshafted type, found among the tribes of Oregon and northern California. The ideas made specially prominent are: FIG. 1. The method of inserting the foreshaft into the end of the shaft. FIG. 2. The attachment of the head to the barb piece by diagonal lashing of sinew and the union of the stone head with the barb piece of bone attached to the foreshaft. FIG. 3. The laying on of the feathering in one example having what is called the "rifling" of the arrow. FIG. 4. The foreshaft before the head is attached, showing especially the neat manner of its union with the shaft. FIG. 5. The painted bands or ribands of the shaftment, called by a variety of names. FIG. 6. The relation of the nock to the pithy wood of the shaft. (PLATE XL, Smithsonian Report, *1893)*

The many years between Bourke's observation and the Laubins' statement more than likely brought adaptations and more efficient construction techniques. Or perhaps the bows familiar to Bourke were used by the Chiricahuas in warfare, whereas the bows the Laubins discussed may have been created later for different purposes.

Bourke's interest also extended to arrowheads. In an effort to determine how quickly an Indian could rearm himself after being stripped of (or losing) his weapons (a question of military significance), Bourke timed an Aravaipa Apache at this work, according to Joseph C. Porter, his biographer. The Indian created four flint arrowheads in an average time of six and one-half minutes each.[23]

Arrows had to be carried carefully. Native Americans created quivers from deer or antelope hides by sewing the skins together in the shape of a long tube. Each quiver had a stick sewn inside all along its length that helped maintain the shape. According to Peckham, native warriors also created wrist guards for themselves made from leather straps to which were fastened "anywhere from six to eighteen bone

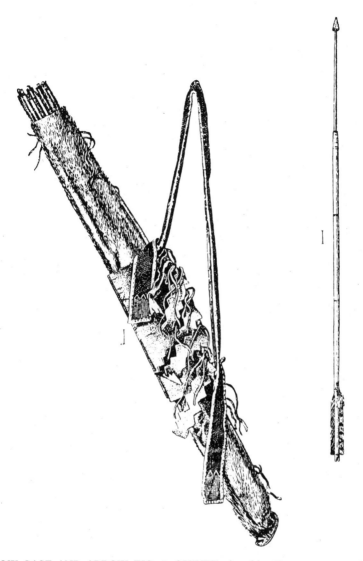

ARROW CASE AND ARROW. FIG. 1. QUIVER, deerskin. Bow case, none. Arrow case, bag with a stiffener of wood attached by means of strings along the seam. About the middle of the quiver is a band of smoked deerskin leather, with a fringe characteristic of the tribe, in which the scallop before mentioned appears. The bandolier is a strip of cotton cloth and blue flannel. Length of quiver, 34 inches. Cat. No. 17331, U.S.N.M. Apache Indians, Athapascan stock, Arizona. Collected by Dr. H. C. Yarrow, U.S. Army. Note.—The arrows accompanying this quiver, of which an example is given, are of the characteristic Apache type, shaft of reed, foreshaft of hardwood, points of iron. The extra length of the quiver is due to the fact that the reed arrows are longer than those with shafts of hardwood. (PLATE LXXVIII, Smithsonian Report, *1893)*

tubes an inch to an inch and one-half long, placed side by side."[24]

Before using the arrows, a decision had to be made about whether to "poison" the tips. At least two methods for this were available. Dr. J. H. Bill, writing in 1862, described a putrefaction process used by Arizona's Hopi Indians to contaminate their arrowheads. They exposed the liver of a small animal to the fangs of a rattlesnake. After venom had been infused, the organ was "removed, wrapped in the animal's skin and buried" for about a week. It was then resurrected, and the points were dipped in the rotting mess. When the projectiles were dry, they were dipped in blood, again dried, and preserved for use. Although the Hopis undoubtedly used this poison, Dr. Bill himself never witnessed the process, and "among some seventy-six cases of arrow wounds received from Nabajoe [sic], Apache, and Utah Indians, we have seen no case of poisoned arrow wound in the human subject, nor have we heard of such a case after careful inquiry."[25]

Dr. John C. DaCosta, in his textbook on surgery, stated that as far as he knew, "the Piutes [sic] were the only tribe of North American Indians [that poisoned their arrows]." Dr. DaCosta cautioned that

> it is particularly important to remove a poisoned arrow at once. After removing a poisoned arrow, if the nature of the poison is known, proper treatment should be applied to antidote the poison. The French Colonial surgeons fill wounds inflicted by poisoned arrows with tannic acid. The same custom is followed by English surgeons in West Africa.[26]

Another person who wrote on this fascinating topic, Virgil Y. Russell, concentrated his descriptions on the types of arrowheads that held the toxins most efficiently. A jagged, serrated-edged iron point was best, he claimed, because the serrations held the poison. His second choice was an arrowhead made on the principle of a fishhook—it penetrated easily but was almost impossible to remove. Russell wrote that Indians "took a piece of fat meat, let a [rattlesnake] bite it many times . . . then the arrow points were put into the poisoned meat and baked. . . . The points were allowed to rust before they were baked in the poison meat. Thus, the poison penetrated deep into the points." Another way Native Americans created deadly poisons for their arrowheads, according to Russell, was to "place a piece of liver on an ant hill and allow the ants to bite it for some time. Then the points were placed into the liver and left there until the liver decayed."[27]

Clearly, the major function of the entire bow-and-arrow system was to propel the arrowhead. Without a point, usually made from chipped stone, bones, antlers, metal, or hardwood, the weapon was virtually functionless. The purpose of the arrowhead was to stun, wound, maim, or kill an animal or enemy. And in order to achieve this purpose, the projectile's tip was pragmatically and specifically crafted from earliest times to meet the needs of its users.

Most primitive tools were made of stone, and flint was more than likely the choice of many early Native Americans for their arrowheads, at least in the Southwest. A bowyer used a striker stone to knock flakes off a larger stone and then, through increasingly refined blows, shaped and honed the flakes to his liking. Some became so sharp that they were literally bladelike;[28] others, especially those crafted to stun, were deliberately blunt.

Many points used by early southwestern natives have been excavated, identified, and named.[29] According to Kenneth Honea, whose pamphlet on early projectiles in the Southwest is a useful source of information, Blanco points, named after the Blanco River in central Texas, were probably among the earliest points used in the Southwest. The few existing specimens of Blanco points, found near the Blanco River and in other parts of Texas and central and southeastern New Mexico, are lanceolate in shape, have a broad midsection and a flattened oval shape, and are about 4 to 6 centimeters long, 2 to 2.5 centimeters wide, and 0.7 to 1 centimeter thick.

Sandia points I, II, and III were named for the general area in which they were found—the Sandia Mountains of Albuquerque, New Mexico. These too are among the oldest dated points. Sandia I points are lanceolate and somewhat asymmetrical, with a shoulder on one side of the stem. They vary in length from about 6 to 9 centimeters, with widths from 2 to 4 centimeters. These lance and dart points were made by direct percussion; the flake scars on their faces are irregular. Sandia II points are similar, but instead of a rounded base they have a straight or slightly concave base. The workmanship is more refined. Sandia III points are similar to Sandia II except that the base is deeply concave and the stem is always vertically fluted.

Still in New Mexico, a treasure was excavated from a site near Clovis that came to be known as Clovis points. The site, at the bottom of a late Pleistocene pond in the eastern New Mexico town close to the west Texas border, included the remains of mammoths and other extinct animals. The same points were later found at other, widely separated sites in Nebraska, Colorado, Arizona, Texas, northern Mexico, California, the East Coast, the Midwest, Alaska, and Canada. The points are symmetrically lanceolate, broadest in the midsection and slightly rounded at the tips. Clovis points have characteristic fluting that usually extends up from the base and about halfway to the tip. More than likely this fluting was achieved by indirect percussion; flakes were made probably by direct percussion. These points range from 3.5 to 14 centimeters in length and from about 2 to 4 centimeters in width.

Folsom points were found in northeast New Mexico, closely associated with the remains of an extinct form of giant late Pleistocene bison. They also are symmetrically lanceolate, broadest at the midsection and fluted on either one or both faces, with the flutes extending upward for almost the entire face. The base is concave, and the average dimensions are 3 to 8 centimeters long, and 1.5 to nearly 3 centimeters wide. Folsom points show careful workmanship, with shaping by either direct or indirect percussion or pressure. The vertical fluting was probably produced by indirect percussion.

Hell Gap points have been found at sites in east-central Wyoming, Montana, Colorado, New Mexico, Arizona, California, Texas, and Canada. The workmanship of these points is cruder than that of the various points uncovered in New Mexico, but Hell Gap points present familiar characteristics. They are lanceolate and have slightly rounded upper lateral edges and tapered lower lateral edges that end in what might be considered a stem. They are 4.5 to 8.8 centimeters long, and 2 to 3 centimeters wide. Flaking on these points was created by direct percussion; basal thinning was by multidirectional flaking. The stem and base were smoothed by grinding.

Milnesand points occur widely in eastern New Mexico and western Texas, as well as in Nebraska, Iowa, Alberta, Saskatchewan, and Alaska. They too are lanceolate, broadest either at the midsection or somewhat above, and have slightly to markedly rounded upper lateral edges and tapering lower edges. These points average approximately 5 to 8 centimeters in length and 2 to nearly 3 centimeters in width. The workmanship is generally fine and was achieved with direct or indirect percussion. The lower lateral edges and bases have been carefully smoothed. Archaeologists have noted the similarity of Milnesand points to Plainview points and believe the two are related. That certainly is possible geographically, since both types were found in the general area of the New Mexico–Texas border.

Plainview points were first discovered at a bison kill site near Plainview in the Texas Panhandle. They are generally lanceolate, with the upper lateral edges slightly rounded on most specimens. The lower lateral edges are usually straight and parallel-sided up to about one-half or three-fourths the distance from the base to the tip. The base varies from slightly rounded to markedly concave. The workmanship is quite fine, and the dimensions are 4.5 to 8 centimeters in length, and 1.8 to 2.8 centimeters in width. Archaeologists believe these points were made about 9,000 to 10,000 years ago.

Midland points, found near Midland, Texas, are contemporaneous with New Mexico's Folsom points, which they greatly resemble, although they are not fluted. The deposit in which they were found, which also included human remains, dates back about 11,000 years. Similar points have been found in other regions of Texas and in central New Mexico. According to Honea, Midland points are quite frequently found together with Folsom points in west Texas and New Mexico.

There is also a group of miscellaneous points that may or may not be part of the mythology of the West and Southwest. According to Towana Spivey, director of the Fort Sill Museum in Oklahoma, Indians made arrow tips from just about anything suitable they could find. When raiders brought back skillets, gun barrels, wagon wheels, and the like, warriors hammered out points from the metals they contained. In the 1800s, according to Spivey, there was a bell maker in Missouri who specialized in making bells to be hung on ox yokes and horse tack. The Indians cut arrowheads from his bells after they were plundered from hapless wagon trains. One story has the merchant perishing from an arrow whose tip had been crafted from one of the bells.[30]

And so, in the West and Southwest as in all other areas of Indian America, the natives used a variety of lance and dart points and ar-

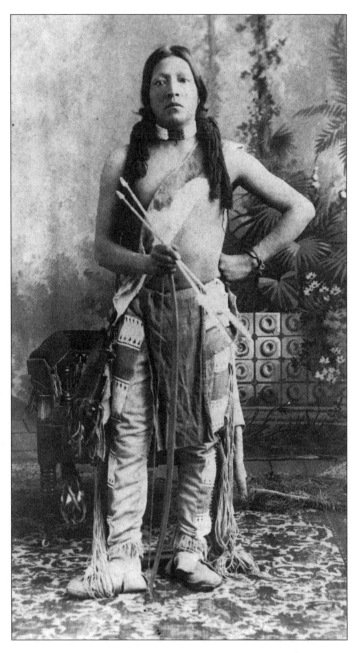

Unidentified young Apache, striking a proud pose with his arrows, ca. 1885. May be Kiowa-Apache. (Photo by Dana B. Chase; courtesy Museum of New Mexico, #110506)

rowheads, all descendants of early man's prototypical points, to kill game and enemies. When the United States Army came on the scene, the indigenous peoples utilized their awesome skills with these deadly weapons to defend the homelands that had been given to them by their Creator.[31] Bows, arrows, and arrowheads—simple implements, some might say—worked for many years to protect the Indians' ways from the white man's will. And these weapons caused injuries so severe that military physicians and others, the surgical heirs (in a manner of speaking) of Cabeza de Vaca and his earlier medical ancestors, the barber-surgeons, found great value in recording and passing on the techniques available at the time to treat arrow wounds.

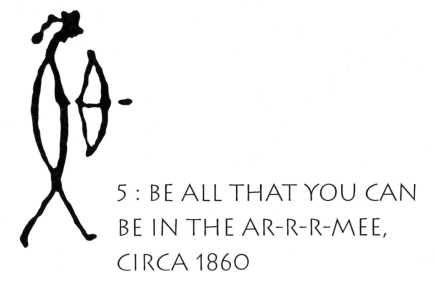

5 : BE ALL THAT YOU CAN BE IN THE AR-R-R-MEE, CIRCA 1860

It is said that Hippocrates, the father of medicine, devoted one of his books to "missiles and the wounds made by them,"[1] but that tome is one of his lost books. Too bad. It certainly would have been a great help in understanding the historical treatment regimens from which later protocols evolved. Indeed, some of Hippocrates' original suggestions, in modified forms, may still be in effect today. With regard to arrow wounds and their remedies, however, almost everything the public (and doctors) knows can be traced back about fifty years or so—to Republic Pictures and other Hollywood motion picture studios.

Movies re-create the chaos and bloodletting that occurred in battles between soldiers and Indians, cowboys and Indians, and Indians and Indians. The finer points of doctoring the injuries received in those battles are usually overlooked in movies, although gross and graphic examples of war injuries are often included. Surely one cannot easily forget the sight of Kevin Costner's leg wound in *Dances with Wolves* or the compassionate military doctor who eventually returned the limb to fairly normal use. Under actual battlefield conditions, of course, the bloody blob would have been lopped off and Costner's adventures, romance, and enlightenment among the Sioux would never have occurred—and all of those touched by the movie (and book) would have been the losers. For reasons I leave unexplored in this book, *Dances with Wolves* awakened, or reawakened, the general public's interest in the American West and its history. Good.

Dr. J. H. Bill, an army physician who practiced in the West and Southwest circa 1860–90, wrote extensively about arrow wounds and recorded detailed descriptions of a broad range of related facts. For instance, Dr. Bill concluded from his observations that arrow wounds healed much quicker in the desert than at sea level. This may seem to be an unimportant conclusion, but to an injured soldier in Arizona and his battlefield surgeon, both worrying about the future of the soldier's wounded limb, Dr. Bill's pronouncement offered hope. Military leaders could also take heart from this information, for the quicker a soldier got back into the fight, the better it was for his unit.

Arrow wounds were not always, or even usually, fatal. For example, Dr. Bill reported the case of Private Martin of the Third Infantry, who was shot in his right leg by an arrow. Lucky for Martin, the arrow passed through the soft tissue and never struck the bone. If it had, Martin's prognosis would have been much less optimistic and Dr. Bill's treatment would have followed a different course. As it was, the surgeon cut into the bleeding wound, sliced a big nerve to still the soldier's agonizing pain, and allowed the wound to heal itself. Private Martin returned to duty on the twenty-eighth day after the injury. Not everyone was so fortunate.

As I have already said, arrows are deliberately designed to ensure maximum physical damage. Further, the way an arrow is released from the bow also influences the type of damage it causes. Spencer L. Rogers described five forms of arrow release used by Native Americans and ranked them according to the power they generated, with the "primary" form being the weakest:

1. Primary: used in the Northwest and Northeast. In this release, the thumb and index finger pinch the arrow neck and pull back the string.

2. Secondary: used in the Southwest, Great Lakes region, and Northeast. In addition to the thumb and index finger, the middle finger also aids in pulling back the string.

3. Tertiary: used in the Great Plains and the Southwest. During this release, the thumb and three fingers draw the string while the arrow is balanced between the thumb and the side of the index finger.

4. Mediterranean: used by Eskimo and in the extreme Southwest. The arrow is held between the index and middle fingers with the string being pulled by the same fingers; the thumb is not used.

5. Mongolian: used in California by one tribe, the Yahi. The thumb alone draws the string, usually with the aid of a ring.[2]

The primary, secondary, and tertiary releases constitute a primitive type of shooting, and the Mediterranean and Mongolian types are more refined forms. Thus, according to Rogers's reasoning, tribes were more or less adept at slaying or wounding according to how they held and released their arrows. Whatever grip they used when shooting arrows, most Native Americans wrapped the stem of the arrowhead with tendons after fitting it snugly into the shaft. On contact with flesh or bone, the sinew was bathed in the victim's body fluids, which caused the wrap to swell and stretch. Thus, when the shaft was tugged or pulled out by the panicked victim, many times the arrowhead, loosened by body fluids (especially copious amounts of blood), slipped easily out of its mooring and remained in the body. Depending on where on the body the arrow struck, muscles might also contract around the arrowhead and hold it so tightly that removing it presented an enormous challenge. In some cases the surgeon had to be both skillful and creative to devise a method of removal. If the arrowhead hit a bone and became stuck, however, nothing but forcible traction and all the strength the physician possessed could remove it.

Army doctors carried special surgical instruments for these circumstances. A wire loop with a long stem could be rigged and inserted into the wound after the physician dilated the wound opening with a bistoury. Splitting muscle and fascia along the arrow's pathway into the flesh, often using only his fingers, the doctor determined the location of the point by probing the immediate area. After that, the wire, the opposite end of which was threaded into an instrument known as Coghill's suture twister, was introduced into the tunnel and shoved closer and closer to the embedded arrowhead. When contact was made, the surgeon carefully manipulated the wire loop so that it encircled the point. After the wire was drawn tight and fastened to the handles of the suture twister, the wire was rocked from side to side as traction was generated by the handles of the instrument. If the wire didn't break, the arrowhead eventually came loose from the bone and could be withdrawn. If the wire broke, the doctor was forced to try again.[3]

Naturally, Native Americans didn't have the medical equipment carried by army physicians, and their technique for removing arrowheads was much more basic—but surprisingly similar. Indians split willow sticks or some similar wood, scraped out the pith, and rounded the ends so they could be inserted to follow the track of the wound. Two sticks were introduced separately, and then both were manipulated so as to reach and cover the point. Then they were withdrawn, together with the point, if the injured person was lucky.[4]

A soldier's arms were the most vulnerable part of his body. Dr. Bill observed that "the upper extremity is oftenest wounded, next comes the abdomen [a favorite target of Indians, who knew well the deadliness of such wounds], next the chest, and next the lower extremity."[5] The head and neck were the least often affected.

Dr. Bill's explanation for the preponderance of arm injuries was that a person could see an arrow flying through the air toward him and instinctively raised his arm to protect his head. All the shooter had to do after that, of course, was aim a little bit lower and hit the same fellow in the chest or abdomen before he could lower his arm. And since an expert native bowman could shoot about six arrows per minute, the soldier on the receiving end ordinarily acquired more than one arrow wound.

Private Robert Nix of Company G, Fourteenth Infantry, was wounded near Camp Lincoln, Arizona Territory, in October 1868. He received a gunshot wound in the upper portion of his left arm, a slight cut from an arrow in the left ear, two flesh wounds from arrows, two arrow wounds in the right knee, one gunshot wound in the right elbow, and another through the bone of the third finger of the right hand. This unlucky soldier was eight hours away from camp and had to get back there riding horseback with a buddy. After arriving and being made comfortable, he suddenly died, not from his wounds but probably of a heart condition that had been previously noted in his medical record.[6]

In the middle 1800s, a Private Bishop was shot in the upper arm, probably because he was protecting his head from an oncoming projectile. The arrow had an iron point that became deeply embedded in the bone. The soldier was in agony. He had lost all motion of his arm and was bleeding profusely and hemorrhaging other body fluids simultaneously. Dr. Bill enlarged the wound, inserted his finger, and determined where the arrowhead had lodged. Next, he introduced forceps into the opening and grabbed the point by its base, but he couldn't move it. Finally, bracing his knees against the patient's chest, he gave a powerful pull, and out it came. If it hadn't been for an assistant standing directly behind him, the doctor would have fallen to the ground, still clasping the instrument that grasped the arrowhead. (This is the stuff of modern animated cartoons.) The patient recovered quite well after being medicated with "evaporating lotions" and fed a diet designed to keep down his fever.

Private James Burridge, a twenty-two-year-old soldier attached to Company C, Fourteenth Infantry, was wounded in a battle with Apaches near Bower's Ranch in the Arizona Territory on November 11, 1867, when an arrow struck his arm approximately two inches above the elbow. By early January of the following year, Burridge knew he had a problem. The arm hadn't healed properly, and a traumatic aneurysm, soft and pulsating and the size of a pigeon's egg, had formed. The military surgeon told Burridge to apply pressure to the area with his fingers and hold the bloody tumor down. One week later, after Burridge had followed the doctor's instructions carefully, the egg was reduced to half the size. By January 18 the mass had practically disappeared. Burridge returned to active duty on January 20, 1868.[7]

In the same battle, forty-five-year-old Private William Hardwick, also of Company C, received arrow wounds in his left thigh and right arm. The arrows penetrated the muscle tissue right up to the bone and lodged there. Assistant Surgeon P. Middleton operated on Hardwick right there on the battlefield, giving the soldier a whiff of chloroform before he enlarged the wounds and removed the arrows. The next day, Private Hardwick was admitted to the post hospital at Camp Whipple. By December 15, both wounds had healed, but the patient had regained only slight use of his leg. Two weeks later he could walk with crutches, and less than a month after that Hardwick was returned to active duty.

Not all cases were as easily handled. Occasionally arrowheads wrapped themselves around bones, making their removal extremely difficult. Dr. Bill recorded a case in which an iron arrowhead had been lodged in a man's thigh for six months. The surgeon who attended the patient soon after the injury occurred removed the arrow's shaft but couldn't extricate the point. Infection set in and produced abscesses, pus, fever, and all the usual complications. The man was near death when Dr. Bill took charge. He found the arrowhead wrapped around the femur. After an extremely bloody dissection, he manipulated the point quite skillfully and eventually loosened it enough to pull it out. The soldier's leg was splinted, compresses and bandages were applied, and he received "proper constitutional treatment." He recovered good use of his leg.

Yet another case concerned a surgeon who was himself wounded in the armpit while fighting Navajos in the Southwest.[8] As was often the case, the shaft came out easily, but the arrowhead remained in the doctor's body for quite some time. He finally consulted another surgeon, who made a T-shaped incision over the scapula and located the point. It was so twisted and bent that a great deal of manipulation was necessary to loosen and remove it. Complications in the form of a hemorrhage occurred twelve hours after the surgery, but the bleeding was controlled and the physician eventually recovered.

In an 1862 article Dr. Bill documented the arrow wounds he had treated during one unspecified period. He compiled the following statistics on injuries to various parts of the body:[9]

Head, 5
Spinal marrow, 1
Neck, 2
Chest, 15
Heart, 2
Abdomen, 21
Upper extremity, 28
Lower extremity, 6

One of the most serious places a soldier could be wounded was in the belly. Vital organs and blood vessels are concentrated in the abdomen, and fatal infection can develop if the intestines are perforated. Abdominal wounds from any weapon were generally fatal in the old West and Southwest before the advent of antibiotics and other medications powerful enough to face down the terrible infections that usually followed. Dr. Bill wrote about twenty-one cases of arrow wounds to the belly suffered during a battle with the Navajos. Seventeen of the injured died: thirteen from peritonitis and four from uncontrollable hemorrhage. Nine of the thirteen men who died from infection had been exposed to the broiling desert sun without water for two days, and none lived to reach the military post. All the men were autopsied, and fecal matter was found floating in their abdominal cavities.

Had any of them survived to reach the post, the surgeon would have begun their treatment by locating the arrowhead and removing it, just as he would have removed a point from a less vulnerable spot. In these and similar cases, Dr. Bill concluded that if the shaft of an arrow had been already removed, there was little chance of finding its head, but he urged that every effort be made to do so nonetheless. When it was possible to find and remove the point, the next step involved suturing the bleeding internal organs and cleaning the interior belly with water containing a little salt and egg serum. Then, outer sutures were placed and, if necessary, moist heat was applied using large bran poultices, taking care not to burn the healing external wound. Dr. Bill recommended that after the primary danger of peritonitis had passed, the patient should be kept in a "horizontal position for a month and fed chiefly on beef, or mutton, or fowl, to which it will be prudent to add some pepsin. Olive oil will keep the bowels in a proper condition."[10] Occasionally light custard and milk were added to the patient's dietary regimen, but there was very little else that could be done to expedite the recovery.

American soldiers might have done better to protect themselves against belly wounds as Mexicans did. On entering a battle with Indians, the soldier from south of the border wrapped a blanket around his midsection so that an arrow, if it hit that area of the body, would be stopped cold by the many folds of cloth. If by some happenstance a missile tore through the protection, it usually didn't enter the deeper regions of the abdomen.

Private Conrad Tragesor of Troop I, Eighth Cavalry, would have benefited from such a belly wrap. He was wounded in a battle with Apaches near Sunflower Valley in the Arizona Territory on March 9, 1870. The arrow entered his left side, damaging the kidney during its progress through his abdomen. He pulled the arrow out, but not the point, and then was transported by military ambulance to Camp McDowell, a distance of thirty miles over a rough, stony, and hilly road. Tragesor made it to the fort but died the next day. The surgeon who conducted the autopsy found that the arrow had passed completely through the kidney, but in ripping out the shaft, the soldier had also accidentally torn out a piece of the kidney approximately one inch long and half an inch thick.[11] Had he left the shaft and point intact, his chances of survival would have been better.

Warriors from some tribes safeguarded themselves against belly wounds by wearing a cuirass, a defensive armor made of animal hides that was wrapped around the torso or positioned in front of the body. Occasionally, the expert Plains Indian horsemen used their steeds as protection, even at a full gallop. One especially dramatic battle took place near Fort Larned, Kansas, in 1862 between Kiowas and Pawnees. Kiowa chief Satamore was leading a charge on horseback when he threw himself to the opposite side of his horse, a feat Kiowas and Comanches could perform with great mastery. As he was preparing to aim and shoot his arrows forward from beneath the horse's belly, Satamore couldn't see that an enemy Pawnee was in hot pursuit and gaining on him from the rear. Shortly after the agile chief slipped over the side of his steed, the Pawnee fired his arrow from just a few paces away. It struck Satamore in the buttock. Unperturbed, and still at full speed, the chief reached one arm around to the back of his body and removed the shaft, leaving the iron point behind. He said, years later, that he had passed some bloody urine right after the battle, but the slice in his butt healed quickly, and in just a few weeks he was able to hunt buffalo without too much discomfort. So he ignored the injury.

Satamore remained at the head of his band for six more years, leading them in warfare and in the hunt. He traveled with his people and conducted all the other activities associated with being a Kiowa leader. In August 1869 Satamore appeared at the Fort Sill, Oklahoma, hospital complaining of great pain in the lower abdomen. After confiding in Assistant Surgeon W. H. Forwood about the previous injury to his behind, he gave the army doctor permission to operate on him. Dr. Forwood and another military physician, Dr. H. S. Kilbourne, opened Satamore's belly and removed a stone from his bladder that weighed approximately two ounces. Postoperatively, the doctors sawed the calculus in half and, sure enough, found what Satamore had known all along: the rusty old arrowhead was at its core.[12]

Speaking of Pawnees, the army had problems with this tribe as well. They were excellent marksmen and especially liked to shoot for the torso. Injuries to this area of the body presented particular challenges on the battlefield. For example, a Private Osborn of the Second Nebraska Cavalry was wounded by eight arrows in a skirmish near the Pawnee Reserve on June 23, 1863. All the arrows were removed except the head of one, which had entered at the outer and lower margin of the right scapula and passed upward and inward through the upper lobe of the right lung or trachea. Despite severe hemorrhaging, Osborn recovered, but he continued to have pain on swallowing and occasionally spit up blood. More than three years later, planning to leave his military career because of disabilities he associated with the arrow wounds, he consulted Dr. J. H. Peabody to be examined for a pension. While examining Osborn, the physician found a small opening over the breastbone. Yes, the arrowhead was resting on that bone, with its tip lying flat against the trachea and esophagus. An artery, the jugular vein, and a group of nerves had grown over the top of the point. Getting a good grip on the foreign body, and carefully manipulating it out from underneath the surrounding vessels and nerves, Dr. Peabody removed the four-inch-long arrowhead without Osborn's shedding a drop of blood. By January 1866 Osborn was totally healed. Dr. Peabody denied his pension.[13]

Evacuating chest wounds in which an arrowhead was embedded in a rib was often made easier (for the surgeon) by "placing a block or pile of books" on the patient's chest.[14] In rib injuries that presented no complications, the object was removed and the wound was closed with collodion dressing, and the suffering soldier was instructed to lie on his wounded side and to eat slowly from a special diet that caused little energy to be expended.[15] Often the man was able to return to active duty.

Private Livingston of the Third Cavalry, for example, was wounded on October 6, 1866, at Fort Stevens, Colorado. An arrow entered the right side of his chest, just grazing the first and second ribs. The soldier carefully removed the arrow, including its point, and stated afterward that a great gush of blood helped ease the missile out of his body. He was taken by military ambulance over a rough mountain road to Fort Garland, Colorado, where he arrived six days later very weak and short of breath. He was successfully treated and returned to duty four months later.[16]

Civilian Salvador Martinez had a different experience. An arrow entered his chest between the fifth and sixth ribs on the right side and exited between the seventh and eighth ribs on the left. When Dr. J. H. Bill saw him, Martinez had already removed the arrow and was vomiting blood. After being hospitalized at Fort Defiance and taking half a grain of sulphate of morphia (morphine) at bedtime, the injured man rallied somewhat. The next morning he was given an enema comprising about half a pint of beef essence and two ounces of wine whey. He threw up again and was given half a grain of morphine. That night Martinez had a terrible time breathing and was in great pain. Dr. Bill opened the wound on the left side and a large quantity of blood, serum, and pus spewed out. The next day he felt better, so two enemas were given. On the third day pneumonia appeared in the right lung and the man complained of stomach pains. Peritonitis was diagnosed and he was given two enemas of sulfate of quinia over a period of twelve hours, along with iced champagne by mouth. The wound in Martinez's left side was discharging prodigiously, and he felt a great deal of pressure over the abdomen. That evening, he had two more enemas and seemed to feel better. Unfortunately, he died sixteen days later, after a very rocky course of treatment. Autopsy revealed a solidified right lung engorged with pus and a left lung with a hole the size of a turkey's egg, also filled with pus. The arrow had wounded the right lung, the left lung, the liver, and the stomach. The latter had healed, but the liver contained an open wound, as did the right lung.

One prominent army officer, who has remained anonymous for more than a century, was wounded in 1881 by a Comanche arrow. According to a verbal report of the incident, delivered before the Buffalo (New York) Medical Club, "The weapon pierced the upper part of the right chest and passed nearly horizontally through the lung, the point

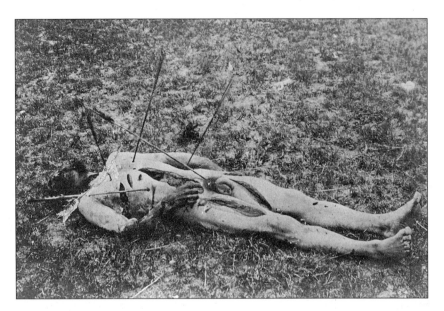

Sergeant Frederick Wyllyams, 7th Cavalry, killed by Cheyennes near Fort Wallace, Kansas, 1867. (Courtesy Fort Sill Museum, Fort Sill, Oklahoma)

protruding at the back between the scapula and the spine." At the wounded officer's request, "a silk handkerchief [!] was fastened to the shaft, which was then pushed through his body, dragging the silk after it through the whole extent of the wound."[17] Believe it or not, this valiant soldier recovered and spent many more years on active duty in the Indian wars.

In 1989, two skeletons were accidentally unearthed at a construction site in the Tucson area. According to Frederick McAninch of the Arizona Historical Society, the bodies had been buried with great care. Both were male and appear to have been Mexicans or Mexican Americans. There were no obvious clues as to how the older man, who was approximately forty to fifty years old, perished, but the other skeleton showed clear signs. That young man was about eighteen to twenty years old and had a chert arrowhead embedded in the ventral (anterior) surface of his sixth left rib. The cause of death was determined to be the arrow wound, which probably pierced the "major vessels above the heart (e.g., aortic or pulmonary arteries)," and "the perforation of the left lung."[18]

If an arrow hit the spinal column, lodged in a vertebra, and stayed there, the situation was immediately critical. Take, for example, poor

Santiago Ortiz, who was shot in the left armpit while visiting Navajo country with a group of his friends. (Whether he was in the employ of the United States Army has not been determined.) He pulled out the shaft of the arrow, but the point remained where it landed—in the fourth dorsal vertebra. By the time Dr. Bill saw him two days later, he had stopped hemorrhaging—helped, of course, by his pals, who plugged the wound with anything they had handy. Try as he may, Dr. Bill couldn't find the offending foreign object, no matter where in the wound's path he probed or how many times he explored the vicinity. Infection ran wild throughout Mr. Ortiz's system, and gallons of empyema (pus) filled his lungs until he died from asphyxiation. The autopsy findings were a surprise: the arrowhead had dislodged itself from the spinal column, moved through the membrane that envelops the lung and lines the chest cavity, and come to rest on the diaphragm.

Others wounded in the spine survived. The Army Medical Museum possesses two remarkable specimens that show the growth of bone around stone arrowheads. One was discovered in 1869 by Acting Assistant Surgeon A. T. Comfort near Fort Wadsworth, Dakota, in the course of exploring ancient Indian mounds. The doctor found a segment of a lumbar vertebra in which a small quartz arrowhead was encysted. "The missile is so overlaid by new osseous [composed of or resembling bone] formation," he reported, "as to prove that the wounded man survived the injury for many months at least."[19]

Injuries to the soft tissues of the upper torso, particularly the vital organs, presented a challenge to battlefield doctors working with limited instruments, medications, and knowledge. A Mexican civilian whose name Dr. Bill didn't know was traveling near Fort Defiance in Navajo country when he was shot with five arrows. All injured the lung, and one passed through the upper border of the liver. Dr. Bill extracted the arrowheads successfully and, after the man stopped bleeding, applied a dressing of muslin soaked in collodion to each of the wounds and put the patient to bed. He was given one grain of morphine. The next morning the man was vomiting, and he was given opium and acetate of lead. By afternoon he complained mightily of pain on the right side and difficulty in breathing. Dr. Bill removed the dressing over the wound that had involved the liver and lung. Blood clots and other fluids were drained, and the patient then said he felt much better. He was told to lie on the side that had the most wounds

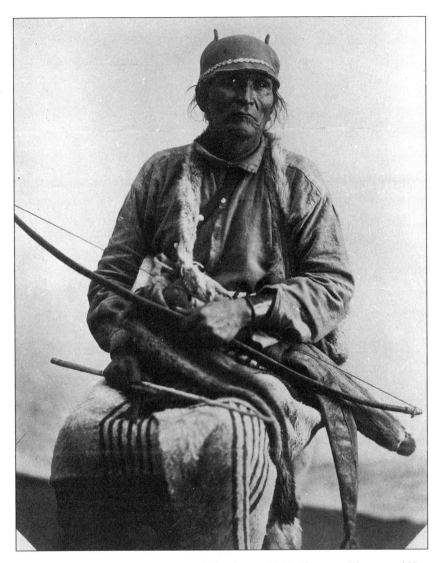

Unidentified Navajo man in Bosque Redondo, ca. 1866. (Courtesy Museum of New Mexico, #38200)

as much as possible. The next day the man vomited a considerable quantity of black, decomposed blood and urinated a very dark fluid. The doctor stopped all medications temporarily until he could get a clearer clinical picture. Lo and behold, this anonymous fellow recovered completely and thereafter went on his way. In six weeks he returned to Fort Defiance to have nasal polyps removed, saying they had bothered him greatly during his recuperation.

Just as an aside, some time before 1893 a Dr. Shufeldt became friendly with a Navajo warrior, an older gray-headed fellow who had participated in many battles where bows and arrows were the only weapons used. The doctor asked the aging fighter to pretend that he was about to kill his worst enemy and give a demonstration using a bow and arrow.

> The old fellow . . . immediately drew one of them at its very head. This is the position he stood in at the time: His left foot was slightly in advance of the right, the bow was firmly seized at its middle with the left hand, while it was held somewhat obliquely, the upper moiety inclining toward the right from the vertical line, and, of course, the lower limb having a corresponding inclination toward the left side. The two spare arrows were held with the bow in the left hand, being confined by the fingers against its right outer aspect. With the right hand he seized the proximal end of the arrow in the string, using the thumb and index finger, at a point fully an inch or more above the notch, and consequently including the feathers. The ring finger bore against the string below this seizure, and its pressure was re-enforced by its being overlapped by the middle digit, the little finger being curled within the palm of the hand . . . the arrow at its head was on the left side of the bow and simply rested on top of his clinched hand. This man wore, in common with all the others who used the bow, a stiff leather bracer, fastened by buckskin strings about his left wrist, the collar being about 2 inches deep, and this . . . was ornamented with silver buttons. He drew the arrow back and forth three or four times without changing the position of his finger or hands. . . . Upon further questioning him, he told me that the Navajoes rarely held their spare arrows in the bow hand, as he now had them, but carried a scabbard (quiver of buckskin) full, in front of them, from which they could be removed with great rapidity while firing.[20]

Neck wounds were generally not fatal unless the larger vessels were hit or the trachea was pinned to the spine by the projectile. Dr. Bill never encountered this type of injury himself, but he cited Conrad the Red, duke of Lorraine, a prominent man in European history who, having removed his helmet at the moment of victory over the Hungarians, was shot in the neck and died quickly.[21]

A simple note by Dr. Bill about arrow wounds to the heart said it all: they were generally fatal, although not always instantaneously so. In one battlefield case, the injured soldier lived five minutes, during which he pulled the shaft from his chest and discarded it. When Dr. Bill arrived at the man's side, he couldn't tell whether an arrow had struck the fatal blow or the enlisted man had been shot with a pistol ball from a comrade's weapon. The entry wound greatly resembled one made by a Colt revolver. In the autopsy, however, the question was answered. An arrow had pierced the top of the soldier's heart, and its tip was lodged in a vertebra.[22]

A more remarkable experience was described by noted author and historian Dan L. Thrapp. On July 27, 1867, frontiersman Harvey Twaddle was rounding up stray mules near Walnut Grove, Arizona, when he was shot in the heart by an arrow. Using a Henry rifle, he killed the Indian who had shot him and a second, and wounded a third; then he chased two mules back to camp. Delirious with fever, he recovered sufficiently to tell what had happened, but succumbed nine days later. Examination after death revealed that a headless arrow had actually penetrated his heart.[23]

The cases presented above are summarized in Dr. Bill's considered and learned opinion regarding the prognosis in cases of arrow wounds:

[It] depends on several circumstances. It is influenced . . . by the nature of the parts wounded. Vessels and intestines are not pushed aside, as they frequently are by bullets, but are laid open; fecal matter may be thus thrown into the peritoneum, or a hemorrhage, sufficient to determine the fatal issue, may take place. . . . Not only have we to consider the blood already lost, but that which is likely to be lost in extracting the missile.

Another variable in the prognosis was the status of the arrow. Ideally, the doctor wanted to remove the entire apparatus intact. Of course, if the point had dislodged from the shaft and its removal was tricky, the victim was in trouble. Dr. Bill also mentioned the general health of the wounded person as an essential component of predicting outcomes, as well as the "immediate importance of the wounded parts to life."[24]

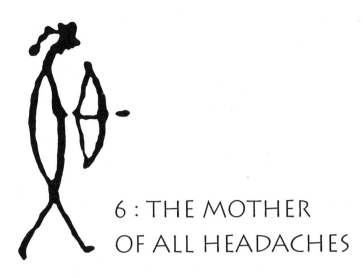

6 : THE MOTHER
OF ALL HEADACHES

The several tribal legends that mention blows to the head leave no doubt that Native Americans considered such injuries to be quite serious. As a matter of fact, one Alaskan Indian tale locates a second heart in the brain.

> The daughter of an Indian chief had been abducted by a bear and carried away to sea. She escaped and finally reached the shore. Out in the water she saw a fisherman in his boat and she called to him to rescue her from the animal. The fisherman touched the gunwales of his canoe with his club, and it was at once on the shore. At this moment the bear and some of his tribe appeared. The fisherman began to fight with the bear but could not land a telling blow. Then the chief's daughter said, "Strike the bear between the eyes, because his heart is there." When the bear was struck on the head, he was killed. The fisherman then took the chief's daughter in his canoe. He proved to be Gonaquet, the spirit of the sea.[1]

Among the Iroquois, invulnerability to head wounds implied supernatural power.

> A giant man-eater by the name of Kahnahchuwahne [He-Big-Kettle] sat by his boiling kettle, beating his drum. The hun-

gry people danced around him, hoping that he would give them some soup. Then he would suddenly seize one of them and eat him. Okwencha [Red Paint], who was standing to one side, then seized his war club. He ran to He-Big-Kettle and struck him on the forehead, but the giant seemed not to notice. After the third blow, the giant said: "It seems to me the mosquitos are biting."[2]

Along with these American Indian legends are records of actual battles between Indian groups that describe face and head injuries. The death of a warrior called Lights-on-the-Cloud is an example. This man, from an unknown Plains tribe,

> obtained a shirt of mail, evidently an heirloom of the Spaniards, against which the flint-headed arrows of his enemies, the Cheyennes, shattered harmlessly. Wielding a large sabre, Lights-on-the-Cloud rode without harm up and down the ranks of his enemy, challenging them to fight. One [Cheyenne], braver than the rest, stood his ground, however, and shot a sacred arrow through [Lights-on-the-Cloud's] eye into the brain, killing him instantly.[3]

In 1854 or thereabouts, a Pawnee killed a Cheyenne, a leader known as Eagle Feather. The unlucky Cheyenne was shot between the eyes with an arrow by the Pawnee, whom he was attempting to strike with his lance.[4]

A Cheyenne legend tells of a boy who became a hero because of a deed involving a bow and arrow. After traveling a long time, the boy, who was named Falling Star, reached camp and went into his grandmother's tent. It was autumn in the northern high country and the weather was very cold. He asked, "Grandmother, why don't you have a fire? I am very cold." The old woman turned to her grandchild and replied, "We cannot get any wood. In the timber lives a Great Owl who kills people whenever they go for wood." Over the objections of his grandmother, the boy took his bow and arrows, a rope, and an ax and started out to look for wood. He found several dead trees and began chopping, all the while keeping an eye out for the owl. Suddenly the great bird appeared and with one giant swoop caught up the boy and put him in its ear. The boy took his bow and one of his arrows and shot the bird in its brain. It fell down dead, and the boy returned to his grandmother—and his tribe—with wood and a hero's status.[5]

While this owl, a prominent figure in Cheyenne mythology, couldn't remove the arrow from its head, human victims of head and face wounds frequently could. Although injuries in this area were often not fatal, it is difficult to imagine a more terrifying situation. The young man from Portland, Oregon, who lost an eye to an arrow while trying to gain admittance to Mountain Men Anonymous (see Chapter 1) is only one among a long list of adventurers—natives and non-natives, civilian and military—who lived to suffer the consequences of their wounds. Others were not so lucky (or unlucky, depending on your perspective). They died.

The Army Medical Museum owns a skull that dates back to approximately 1871 and shows evidence of a facial injury. The arrow had entered just above the soldier's cheekbone, passed inward, and penetrated the brain. The shaft of the arrow had apparently been removed, leaving the point deeply embedded, hidden and hooked under the cheekbone. Conjecture in this case is that the surgeon would have had to cut away a portion of the cheekbone in order to expose enough of the arrowhead to remove it with forceps and that he decided not to undertake such a procedure. According to the appearance of the skull, this soldier lived about a month with the arrowhead in his cheekbone,[6] plenty of time for the area to become contaminated by microbes of the mouth, nose, and skin. A raging infection probably resulted and was the cause of death.

Another specimen in the same museum, a Sioux Indian's skull, was found near Camp Lewis, Montana Territory, in 1876. An iron arrowhead had penetrated the skull and is still lodged there, bent, perhaps by the victim's headfirst fall to the ground.[7]

In 1869 the Smithsonian Institution contributed the skull of a California Indian to the Army Medical Museum. The man had been wounded by a long arrow point that penetrated the left eye and entered the sinus cavity. From appearances, the wound was not mortal; death came from some other cause, possibly infection.

The skull of a middle-aged Indian male found near Buena Vista Lake in the San Joaquin Valley indicates that he was shot in the right eye by an arrow as he was coming forward in a stooped position, probably stumbling as a result of other arrow wounds. The shaft passed through his eye and entered the nasal cavities. He fell finally and was killed by subsequent blows to the face and head, or so his other skull wounds suggest. Excavations of Indian burials in Sacramento County, California, revealed one skull in which a chert arrow point entered the nose, traveled downward and to the right, and came to rest after it penetrated the hard palate.

An incredible story was reported by Dr. C. C. Gray, an army surgeon assigned to the Dakotas in the late 1860s. Dr. Gray wrote that Private John Krumholz of Company H, Twenty-second Infantry, was wounded at Fort Sully, Dakota, on June 3, 1869, by an arrow that entered his left eye and penetrated the skull for two inches. The soldier was admitted to the fort's hospital the same day. After he was anesthetized with chloroform, an operation was begun to remove the point. Surgeons sawed nearly all the way through his skull with a Hey's saw until they reached the arrowhead, which they removed. Krumholz's postoperative care consisted of rest, a diet low in calories, elevation of the head, applications of cold to the operative site, and saline cathartics. This soldier returned to active duty four days later, June 7, 1869![8]

One particular facial wound reported by Dr. J. H. Bill is typical of many others. A spear-shaped iron point, two and three quarters inches long, entered a soldier's face just a little below the left eye socket and was almost completely embedded in bone; only the stem of the arrowhead protruded into the flesh. The post surgeon wasted no time in trying to extract the foreign body with forceps, but after two hours of probing and pulling he finally gave up. The man remained alive and was sent to St. Louis, where he arrived five weeks after the injury and was seen by Dr. Bill. The left side of his face was swollen, and the entry wound had healed over. Pus was flowing from one of his nostrils. Dr. Bill cut open the area where the arrowhead had initially entered the face and tried to remove the point himself. He failed at first but, after using several different instruments, eventually succeeded. A large amount of bleeding immediately occurred but was stopped by rest, cold, opium, plugging, and bandaging. Soon the patient was able to move around easily and was discharged.

On a later visit to Dr. Bill's office, the soldier complained of stiffness and inability to open his jaws as widely as usual. Dr. Bill determined that this minor disability was due to thickening of certain tissues from the infection, and his advice to the patient was to gently practice opening and closing his mouth. Less than an hour after this exercise began, the man's entire cheek became hot, swollen, and painful, and renewed bleeding occurred. Dr. Bill incised the inside of the soldier's mouth, the cheek, and the neck to allow the discharge of large grumous clots.[9]

The patient hemorrhaged for the next three nights, usually beginning at midnight, oddly, until the physician decided to tie off the carotid artery. This operation was done by candlelight, two months after the man was originally injured. The operation was successful, the bleeding never recurred, and the patient recovered completely.[10]

Private William Drum of the Fourteenth Infantry was wounded in a fight with Apaches on November 11, 1867. One arrow entered the left side of his face and passed along the lower border of the eye socket to within half an inch of his nose. Eight days later the arrowhead was cut out, and less than a month after that, on December 3, he returned to duty.

Whether the wounds were not as bad as they sound, the men were so physically fit that they recuperated quickly, or the army desperately needed soldiers to fight Indians, it seems that many enlisted men who suffered facial wounds were back on the battlefield sooner rather than later. Skull injuries, however, presented different circumstances.

Dr. Bill, the expert on arrow wounds of the head, considered skull injuries less threatening than injuries to other areas. In an offhand, casual statement, the physician declared, "An arrow, unless it strikes at a short range, or perpendicularly to the skull, will usually glance off, making a scalp wound—a wound here requiring no particular notice, as it presents nothing peculiar." But then, in the next breath (so to speak),[11] the doctor became quite serious in his discussion of an arrow wound to the eye socket and a detailed description of what happens when an arrow strikes and penetrates the skull. According to Dr. Bill, when the point enters the skull, it creates a narrow slice in the bone that is roughly the size and shape of the arrowhead. Additionally, however, fracture lines or cracks extend from both ends of the wound

over a distance proportional to the momentum which the arrow possessed. In its passage through the outer table [the exterior skull], the arrow-head loses its momentum and strikes the inner table with a greatly reduced velocity, a velocity not sufficient to allow the arrow-head to penetrate it and pass into the substance of the brain; but enough to cause a scale of the inner table to be fractured off; and whilst still sticking to the point of the arrow-head, to be slightly driven upon (seldom into) the brain itself.[12]

If a soldier who received this type of wound was being watched over by his guardian angel, and if conditions were exactly right, he had a prayer of surviving—provided, of course, that he wasn't dead when he hit the ground. The presence of a surgeon nearby who could reach him quickly before the enemy arrived to finish him off would have been especially fortuitous. The battlefield doctor followed a rather different procedure when removing an arrow from the head. Instead of yanking on the arrowhead and using brute force to pull it out, the doctor used gentle traction. Rocking the missile back and forth and dislodging it slowly from the soldier's head ensured that the least amount of bone and brain matter would be withdrawn when the foreign body was at last released. Assuming that the operation was successful and that bleeding was immediately controlled, the next step was to prevent infection. Croton oil (chloral hydrate, an antispasmodic) was applied, and the wound was closed with collodion. The last procedures included shaving the head and applying cold compresses. If abscesses formed, it was necessary to drill into the skull to release the pressure. Dr. Bill believed that these cases almost always ended in death.

In one remarkable example, a man named Miguel, a post guide at Fort Union, New Mexico, was hit by the arrow of a Ute Indian. The arrow stuck in the back of his skull. In a fit of frenzy, Miguel yanked on the shaft and removed it. Dr. Bill created traction on the point, and after some minutes it easily slid out of the man's head. Miguel turned over, sneezed, got up off the ground, thanked the physician, and walked away. The next day he complained of headache. His face was flushed, his eyes bulged, and his pulse was fast and irregular. The doctor shaved Miguel's head and applied croton oil and cold compresses. Miguel became delirious, and Dr. Bill deliberately bled him until he fainted, thus abruptly interrupting his hallucinations—but only temporarily. That night Miguel went into a frenzy again and had to be bled again. Clearly, Dr. Bill had the right answer, for the next morning the patient was much better. He recovered completely in three weeks and was back at his job at the post.

Southwest of Fort Union lay the Arizona Territory and Fort McDowell. In the spring of 1866, Company B of the Third Battalion, Fourteenth Infantry, was in the area protecting settlers and other civilians from Apaches. Private Andrew Snowden was en route from Maricopa Wells to Fort Goodwin, in the same part of the country, when he was struck in the back of the head by an arrow on March 22. It penetrated his skull. He turned back to Maricopa Wells, a journey lasting nine days from the time he was wounded. He arrived weak and fatigued, but coherent. Along the way he had pulled out the shaft, but the arrowhead remained. Ten days later he lost his appetite, became nauseated, and appeared dull and stupid. Private Snowden was transported on a hay wagon to see Dr. Charles Smart at Salt River, some thirty miles away. Dr. Smart examined the man and found his lucidity and intelligence much impaired. Snowden couldn't even remember his name, much less answer any other questions clearly. He vomited persistently. On April 19 the soldier was admitted to an army hospital where he was given an enema, his head was shaved, and cold dressings were applied to his skull. During the day he lapsed into a deeper stupor, but the vomiting ceased. As there were no results from the first enema, another one was given the next day. At this time Snowden's head wound began oozing through its scar, so it was cut, enlarged, and a probe introduced into the opening. Dr. Smart located the iron point inside the man's head and removed it. During the entire procedure, Snowden lay quietly, but afterward he occasionally burst into wild screams. Postoperatively, he appeared to be paralyzed on the right side and couldn't eat. He urinated normally, but still didn't move his bowels. Enemas were continually administered with no results. By April 30, Snowden appeared to be much better. He was eating, could answer questions, and remembered his name. His head wound was healing well. Although there is no note of it in the case history, apparently his bowels finally moved.

On May 7, Snowden took a bad turn. Fever developed, and he had a restless night. By the next day he had a headache and was sick to his stomach. Dr. Smart ordered an enema and cold compresses to the head. By May 11, his muscles were involuntarily trembling. Unconsciousness set in on the morning of May 13, and Snowden died that afternoon.

An autopsy performed seven hours after death showed a scar on the back and left side of Snowden's scalp. The slit in the skull caused by the arrowhead had been filled in with recently formed soft tissue, a normal occurrence, but the brain tissue in the area where the point had been lodged was softened and disorganized. Dr. Smart reported that the track made by the arrowhead was filled with thick pus that had seeped and spread to various parts of the brain. No other organs were examined.[13]

Assistant Surgeon W. M. Notson described the case of Private Martin W— of Company E, Fourth Cavalry, who was on duty as one of the stage guards on the mail run from Fort Chadbourne to Fort Concho, Texas, when he was struck by a Comanche's iron-tipped arrow. The arrow entered his skull just above and behind the left ear and penetrated to a depth of an inch or more. He bled deep inside the skull and died quickly. At some later time, the man's head, with the arrowhead still lodged in the bone, was forwarded to the Army Medical Museum.[14]

An unusual situation, also recorded by Dr. Notson, began when arrow wounds and bullet injuries were sustained by civilians in a battle with Indians on September 1, 1870, near the Pecos River in Texas. One man in the party was killed, another escaped, and Dr. Notson's patient received an arrow wound to the head and three gunshot flesh wounds. For seven days the injured man traveled—on foot, by wagon, and by stagecoach—to Fort Concho, where he was seen by the doctor and admitted to the post hospital. He complained only of weariness from his ride and some slight soreness from the gunshot wounds in his arm, chest, and leg. He appeared to almost disregard the arrow wound on the side of his head. On the fourth day after admission the gunshot wounds appeared to be healing, but fever had developed. A special diet was ordered for the man, and aromatic spirits of ammonia were given in small doses. By the sixth night after admission, cerebral symptoms appeared and the patient became violent. He was given chloral hydrate to relax him. Two days later, Acting Assistant Surgeon

C. W. Knight reopened the wound in the man's temple but was unable to remove the arrowhead. The patient died on September 19. The autopsy revealed the point to be about half an inch from the external wound and surrounded by pus, which obviously was the result of infection and the cause of death.[15]

Dr. Bill, in a classic medical paper, warned that

> the immediate danger in arrow wounds of the skull is from internal hemorrhage. . . . Encephalitis is the secondary danger to which the victims of arrow wounds of the skull are exposed. If the arrow head is removed, this inflammation will usually not be serious, and will yield to purgatives, ice, aconite,[16] and rest. But if the arrowhead is not removed, the irritation will produce abscess, which will probably prove fatal.[17]

Most of the directions for treating arrow wounds of the face and head were meant to deal with a single arrow wound. Yet, skulls with more than one embedded point have been unearthed, although rarely. For example, Cyril B. Courville reported that Acting Assistant Surgeon H. C. Yarrow found the skull of a California Indian near Santa Barbara with two arrowheads protruding from the rear. Courville hypothesized that the victim might have been a medicine man, possibly from the Chumash tribe, who failed to heal too many patients. Among some tribes, the surviving relatives of dead patients were allowed to kill an unsuccessful healer. Arrows were often the weapon of choice. "Usually," declared Courville, "such arrows were directed at the body, but it is possible that the head was not exempt as a target."[18]

His in-depth study of head injuries led Courville to agree with Dr. Bill, who had concluded years earlier that arrow wounds themselves of the face and skull need not be fatal. In many instances, it was the infection following the injury that was life threatening. "Meningitis," wrote Courville, "or other intracranial infections may have caused the death of some of those who survived the immediate impact. On the other hand," he added, "it must be recognized that the cranial wound was not necessarily the only one present."[19]

It was sometimes necessary to enter a wounded man's skull in order to remove the foreign body. Many times, forceps and other instruments were useless because of the location of the arrowhead, the resistance it presented, or other extenuating circumstances. In those situations, and in several others involving tribal beliefs about organic ailments, there were two choices: surrender the individual to the fates by not intervening, or undertake a procedure known as trephining—opening the skull. Battlefield surgeons had a variety of instruments designed to accomplish that task, but the native peoples used a sharp, bladed stone, a stone drill, or a sawlike implement fashioned from iron.

Either way, it is a chilling thought.

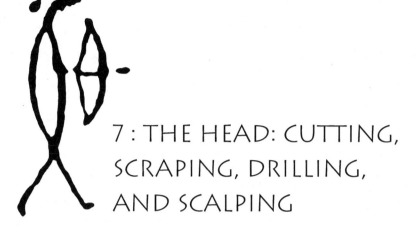

7 : THE HEAD: CUTTING, SCRAPING, DRILLING, AND SCALPING

On the western American frontier, head injuries from arrows were often extremely grave, regardless of whether the wounded were American Indians or U.S. Army soldiers. Head wounds required immediate attention, not only because of their obvious seriousness but also because infection was virtually guaranteed to follow. A head wound was generally contaminated by skin, hair, slivers of bone, and whatever organic matter had been smeared on the arrowhead. Severe hemorrhaging was always present, blood clots often formed, and paralysis could be a complication.[1] Skull fractures frequently accompanied the wound and produced their own tier of symptoms, further complicating the medical picture.

If the injured man was a soldier, a bold army physician might give skull surgery a try on the battlefield, despite having learned in medical school that this type of operation was so risky that it was extremely undesirable under any circumstances. For example, Professor Dudley of Lexington, Kentucky, published an article in 1828 in which he detailed the particulars of only five cases that involved opening the head. No mortality statistics were offered. Dr. J. T. Gilmore of Mobile, Alabama, wrote in the middle 1800s that he entered the skulls of five patients. Three were cured of their problems; two died. Most of the procedures were performed to treat epilepsy and were considered to be very dangerous for the patient.[2]

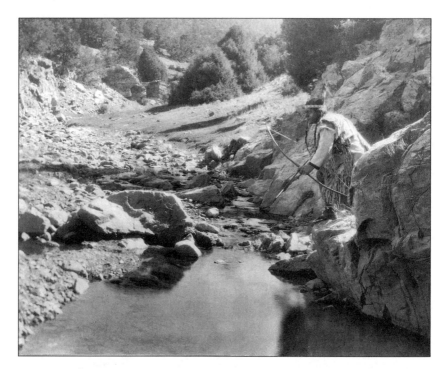

Oskenonton, Mohawk singer at river's edge in New Mexico, ca. 1925. Singers were often holy people and medicine men. (Photo by Guy C. Cross; courtesy Museum of New Mexico, #119181)

But cutting, scraping, or drilling the skull to produce an entryway into the head was routine among certain indigenous peoples, especially in South America.[3] Occasionally a wounded warrior's head had to be opened to remove an arrowhead or other object that had become embedded in the skull case or, worse, directly in the brain matter. A bad fall might result in a smashed skull. In that case, the bits and pieces of shattered bone were located inside the head by a shaman's probing finger, gingerly grasped with homemade instruments, and lifted out through the opening. If an individual suffered from seizures that were thought to be the result of supernatural affliction or bewitchment, traditional surgeons knew exactly what type of opening to make with their tools so that the unearthly force(s) causing the ailment could easily escape.

The native healers who treated medical ailments and performed general surgery on tribal members had remarkable confidence in their ability to cure. Their obvious self-assurance was based on and accompanied by a studied, practical, and extensive knowledge of human anatomy, often dating back to youth or even childhood. Unlike formally educated Western physicians, many shamans became practitioners through a vision received from the spirit world or through a direct message from the Creator. Honored and respected in their village or community, these shamans, male or female, had great legitimacy in the eyes of their relatives and friends. They built their reputations and enhanced their credibility with each patient they were able to help. The healers knew which medicinal plants promoted knitting of a broken leg, for example, and which cured earache. They cleaned wounds with willow and stopped hemorrhages with spiderwebs or scrapings from a tanned skin. They cut out infected flesh and scraped bones with stone or obsidian knives, opened abscesses, and removed arrowheads. They were familiar with the effects of narcotics such as coca, the daturas, and tobacco.

Physician and writer Leonard Freeman believed the Pueblo Indians of New Mexico and Arizona "obtained unconsciousness and analgesia by the administration in heroic doses of a compound of stramonium obtained from the jimson weed." Other North American Indians

are said to have had a crude method of producing local anesthesia by means of tying tightly about the part a strip of cloth or bark impregnated with moistened wood ashes. After a short time the benumbing effects of the lye coming from the wet ashes rendered a fairly painless operation possible.[4]

But in tribes from British Columbia to South America, only the most powerful among the native doctors had the courage to saw open someone's skull and operate on the brain. Europeans called this procedure "trephining," or "trepanation."[5] The instrument used to enter the head was called a "trephine," or in some cases a "trepan." Interestingly, geology and geography both influenced the surgical tools that were used for the procedure. North of Mexico, the native surgeon's instruments were almost always made of flint. Farther south, the Aztecs and Incas used copper knives. The Aztecs also had unique knives made by springing flakes from a core of obsidian. They were so sharp and so effective that the men even shaved with them. Or so 'tis said. In the United States, some California Indians also used flint and obsidian knives. "Certainly," concluded Robert Moes, "these were used in opening abcesses [*sic*] and in removing arrowheads imbedded during the occasional internecine forages."[6]

Aside from treating head injuries received in fights, battles, or accidents, there were also other reasons why apparently peaceful individuals attempted to scrape, saw, cut, bore a series of holes into, or otherwise enter the cranial vault of other human beings. In Europe, for example, trephining was performed on perfectly healthy people to obtain amulets. Reported T. D. Stewart, "These round pieces of skull, often polished and sometimes perforated for suspension, have been found in burials [in Europe] and sometimes accompanying surgically opened skulls." Why? Possibly "to ward off future trouble from trauma. . . . [Or it] may have been an extension of a surgical procedure from therapy to prophylaxis."[7] So the lucky individual who survived the skull surgery had a good luck charm! C. B. Cosgrove concurred with Stewart, stating that although trephining was initially performed postmortem, it might also be conducted by shamans on living captives to acquire a fetish of greater power.[8] Sometimes, when pieces of the skull had been removed, the openings were closed with artificial covers such as custom-sized plates carved from gourds.

Primitive trephining was also a prophylactic measure in ailments such as headaches, dementia, and epilepsy, in which case it was performed to allow the evil spirits inside the patient's head to escape.[9] Excavated skeletons in Peru reveal that shamans there even operated on children. The young skulls show no evidence of trauma that would have required trephining, so the operation must have been performed for supernatural reasons. Whether death occurred as a result of the tremendously dangerous operation could not be determined from an examination of the bones.

The Tello collection at Harvard University's Peabody Museum has the skulls of four children close to the age of six years and eleven skulls of twelve-year-olds. Signs of fractures that could have been responsible for the trephining are evident in seven of these. One child's skull shows the first molars just beginning to erupt. It is chilling to imagine that a shaman, possibly a relative of the child, opened the youngster's head with all the best intentions of curing an ailment, only to later watch the child die, possibly because of the surgery.

These days physicians rarely perform even routine surgery on their friends or loved ones, much less operate on their brains, but surgeons on the western frontier, Indian or non-Indian, often had to attempt brain surgery. There was no other choice. Before bows and arrows appeared, the main weapons of defense and offense were slings, clubs, and other hand-held instruments that could easily bash in an enemy's head. No doubt there were many injuries after battles that called for intervention from the tribe's trusted doctor. Also, the rugged country that some Native Americans called home surely caused falls that resulted in head injuries. The group's healer would have helped the accident victim by employing every means necessary, even opening the skull to relieve distress.

Occasionally, even though obvious injuries were lacking, some North American tribal members, like their South American counterparts, needed trephining to let evil spirits escape. As a matter of fact, many of the skull operations may have been performed to treat ailments caused by magic—or so skulls obtained in the course of anthropological excavations seem to indicate. For example, Carl Lumholtz conducted an expedition into Mexico during the years 1894–97 for the American Museum of Natural History. An old Tarahumara Indian showed him a cave in which skeletons had rested for as long as the elder could remember. Lumholtz and a partner removed two great heaps of stones piled in front of the cave's entrance and entered to find the bones of two women, possibly dead for centuries. The skulls were intact, and one contained "some animal matter," was "fatty to touch," and retained "some odor." The skull showed no "deformities or fractures" and there were "no traces of any injury," Lumholtz wrote.[10] This woman had a round opening a little larger than a dime on the left side of the top of her head, an area of easy access that involved comparatively little danger. According to the examiners, the hole was made several years before her death, probably by a flint tool. The second skull was practically identical to the first with regard to the size of the wound, its position on the skull, and the fact that there was no discernible evidence of an injury that would justify trephining. The second woman seemed also to have survived for quite some time postoperatively. The only difference between the two skulls was that the second had lost all soft tissue and had no aroma.

As to the quality of ancient skull surgery in general, Freeman observed that "most of the trephining operations in America do not seem to have been done very skillfully. They were crude jobs with crude

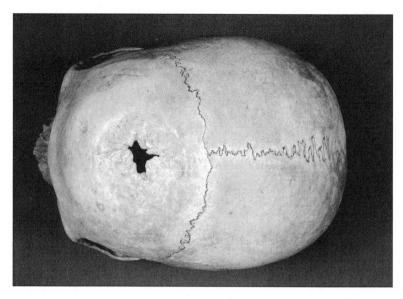

Healed trephination of frontal squama (5.0 cm. in diameter). (Courtesy San Diego Museum of Man)

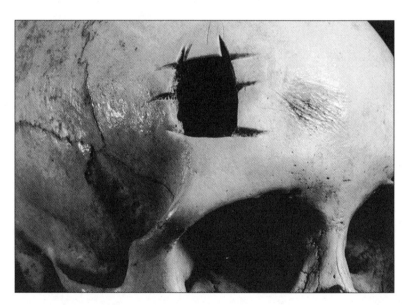

Frontal-right rectangular trephination (approx. 2.2 x 1.8 cm. straight cutting) of adult-female skull with no evidence of healing. Note 1.8 x 1.4 cm.-scraped area on right. (Courtesy San Diego Museum of Man)

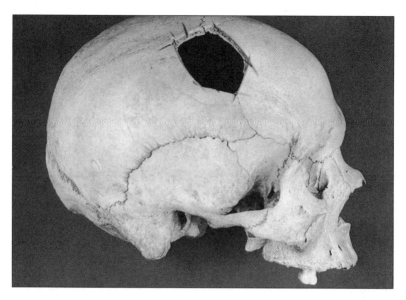

Lateral-right trephination (approx. 4.4 x 3.2 cm. straight cutting) of adult-male skull with no evidence of healing. Separated coronal suture may represent previous trauma. (Courtesy San Diego Museum of Man)

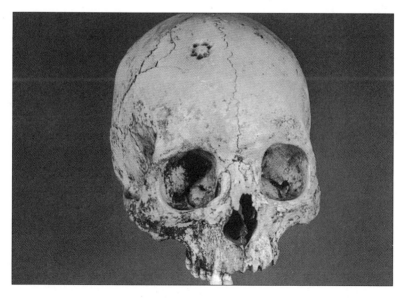

Incomplete trepanation (circle of drill holes approx. 1.6 x 1.5 cm.) on frontal squama. Fracture, as seen on upper left, may have prompted the trephination. (Courtesy San Diego Museum of Man)

tools that often slipped during the laborious process, as shown by scratches on the adjacent parts of the skull." Freeman, a doctor himself, described one method of entering the head—scraping—as a slow process ordinarily accomplished by wearing away the bone with a simple to-and-fro motion of the trephine as the patient sat with his back to the surgeon, his head between the physician's knees.[11]

Aleš Hrdlička identified several other methods used to enter the skull, including trimming, crisscross sawing or cutting, circular or oval cutting, and drilling. "Scraping was employed . . . to remove pressure on the brain. . . . A more frequently employed method was that of sawing . . . through the bone and prying out pieces. . . . Cutting represented the highest form of the art," stated Hrdlička. Drilling produced a number of holes around the section to be removed. The holes were connected by sawing, and the piece of skull was eventually pried out by this more laborious method. Surprisingly, if the patient didn't succumb immediately, the operation was usually followed by normal healing, "without the bones showing any signs of inflammation or suppuration," because, Hrdlička believed, "the Native surgeons doubtless had knowledge of liquids and powders that acted as antiseptics,"[12] and, needless to say, anesthetics. Harry L. Shapiro, an anthropologist, identified another technique as "folding back the skin and laying bare the skull, [then] the desired section was marked out and removed by deep intersection incisions."[13]

Spencer L. Rogers identified three methods of trephining:

> First, a sharp edged implement may be applied as a scraper or plane until enough thickness of the core is removed to produce an opening. Secondly, an implement may be used as a knife or saw in cutting a groove around a central core of bone which it is desired to remove. Thirdly, a pointed instrument may be rotated as an auger or drill and in this way a small hole may be produced.[14]

In his opinion, scraping—with thick quartz flakes, for example— was used only up to a certain point. After that, the surgical method of choice became sawing, which produced grooves around the area that had been scraped. The "saws" were often serrated obsidian flakes. Cutting into the head was the next step, usually with smaller and sharper flakes than those used for sawing. When drilling a series of small holes in the skull was the preferred approach, these holes were later merged into a circular groove by breaking down the walls in between the holes. "A drill of flint or other hard stone would be necessary for this type of operation," Rogers concluded.[15]

According to Freeman, the shape of the opening in excavated skulls is usually "square or oblong, although sometimes round or oval." The square opening is commonest in South American skulls. This type of hole was made by first cutting four rectangular intersecting grooves not quite through the bone to the membrane that encases the brain and then loosening the piece of skull, which was carefully pried out.

And what of the poor patient while all this was going on? Was he or she conscious? No one knows, although Freeman believed that some sort of anesthetic was used by at least one group of natives—the Pueblo Indians of New Mexico and Arizona.[16] Whether Freeman meant that the Pueblo Indians practiced trephining or he was referring to the use of plant narcotics in treating general injuries is not known. If the Puebloans did perform skull surgery, they were among only a few North American Indians who did so.

According to Hrdlička, the U.S. National Museum has more than a hundred skulls from Peru that show evidence of trepanation or related surgical procedures. Other important collections of skulls can be found in the American Museum of Natural History in New York, at Harvard, and in Lima, Peru.[17] Hrdlička examined and photographed many of these skulls and carefully noted their appearance. If no wound was visible, he believed the reason for the trephining to be nonmedical. It is not unusual to find two to five separate trephinings in the same skull, representing repeated operations for reasons obviously not related to violence. At least one skull in a collection Hrdlička viewed had an opening so large that plugs had to be used to prevent herniation of the brain. Examples of the materials used to make these "stoppers" include gourds, shells, and even beaten silver. Several skulls with such stoppers are in the U.S. National Museum's collection, and they show that the patient survived the operation long enough to grow scar tissue and new bone.

The survival rate among patients who underwent trephining in the latter half of the nineteenth century was about 50 percent,[18] and the results of the brain surgery were often quite good, surprisingly so given the circumstances. Many of the specimens Hrdlička examined seemed to indicate that the individual survived for many years after the surgery, based, among other criteria, on evidence of new bone growth around the opening.

Rogers examined fifty-nine skulls from the Hrdlička collection housed in the San Diego Museum that exhibited varying degrees of healing. Thirteen showed no signs of bone recovery, in nine there were slight indications of new bone growth, and in thirty-seven the degree of healing was advanced. Within the last category, two types of bone regeneration occurred: spicules (spikelike fragments of bone) growing from the edges toward the center of the skull wound, and a thickening or thin shelf forming from the inside of the trepanation upward toward the outer aspect of the wound.

Rogers's conclusion is particularly interesting because at the time he wrote the article, in 1938, there was some dispute among members of the medical community about whether new bone growth was even possible after pieces of skull had been removed. An Associated Press item that originated in Atlanta and was published in nationwide newspapers in 1993 indicates that the issue is still somewhat in doubt. Headlined "Skull Reshaping Gives Kids Second Chance," the piece tells an incredible tale of modern skull surgery. An ailment called sagittal synostosis, which occurs about once in every fifteen hundred births, causes the skull to grow in a banana shape. According to the news release, the condition can be corrected fairly simply in infants because their skull bones haven't hardened yet.

This dramatic operation is a giant step forward from the surgical procedure used to reshape children's heads more than twenty years ago, when "the most common procedure consisted of breaking up the skull and teaching relatives to pound on it daily until it molded into a sphere," said Dr. Harold Rekate, chief of pediatric neurosurgery at Barrow Neurological Institute in Phoenix, Arizona. A colleague, Dr. Arno Fried, chief of pediatric neurosurgery at Brown University, added, "We have found that we can do more and more and the healing will be OK and the bone will grow back together."[19]

One aspect of skull surgery, however, hasn't changed much in the last five hundred years. The very first step in trephining, whether done with obsidian blades by native physicians under primitive conditions, on the warring frontier in the 1800s, or in a sterile, high-tech operating room, is to cut a flap of the scalp and peel it back in order to reach the skull to begin the process. Kind of like scalping.

Regardless of whether they killed an enemy with an arrow to the head, some Native American tribes did practice scalping. Tearing a piece of the head and hair from an enemy was, to certain natives, a culturally sanctioned expression of machismo.[20] Where this gruesome practice was first practiced on the North American continent is a matter of speculation. Dr. Erwin H. Ackerknecht believed that Europeans introduced scalping to the natives. Wrote Ackerknecht in 1944, "Scalping in the form to which we are accustomed and in its extraordinary extension was bred only by the white intruders in North America." He later quoted James Mooney, "one of the greatest students of the American Indian and his history," who said that "mutilation was common and scalping (by the white) was the rule down to the end of the war of 1812, and has been practised more or less in almost every Indian war down to the latest."[21]

Worldwide, scalping is an ancient form of mutilation of the fallen enemy practiced because it provided proof of a warrior's prowess to members of his community. Herodotus (484–425 B.C.) described scalping by the Scythians, a nomadic Iranian people. The second book of the Maccabees, from the Apocrypha, records the warfare of the Jews and describes scalping as being a practice of Persian troops. The ancient Germanic code of the Visigoths contains references to scalping as a rite. Anglo-Saxons and Franks scalped their enemies in about 879 A.D. One of the first evidences of scalping by Native Americans was reported by Francisco de Garay, the Spanish administrator of Mexico, in 1520. More records of Indian scalping come from 1534–36 in an account by the French navigator Jacques Cartier, who described how the Huron Indians dried and stretched the scalps of their enemies on small wooden hoops. And J. Wesley Powell's detailed narrative of Spanish-Zuni history in the Southwest includes a description of a 1628 massacre during which Franciscan friars Martin de Arvide and Letrado were killed, mutilated, and scalped.[22]

Hans H. Reese quoted Catlin's description of a method of taking scalps that seems to be rather generalized:

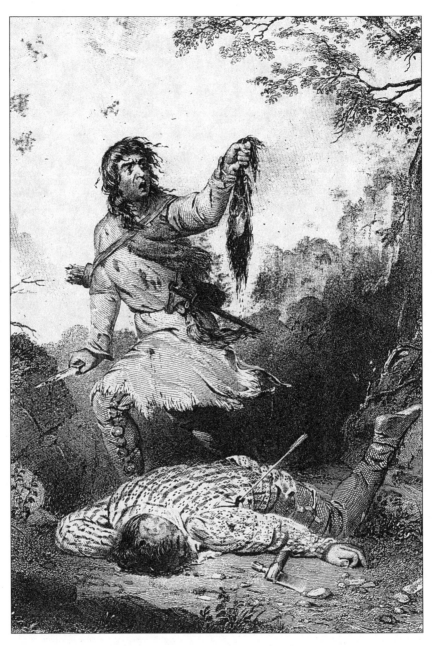

"Death Whoop," drawing depicting a scalping. Careful attention to detail is apparent in blood dripping from hair, blood at arrow's wound. (From H. R. Schoolcraft, History of the Indian Tribes of the United States: Their Present Condition and Prospects and a Sketch of Their Ancient Status.)

The custom practiced by all the North American Indians is done when an enemy is killed in battle, by grasping the left hand into the hair on the crown of the head, and passing the scalp knife around through the skin, tearing off a piece of the skin with the hair, as large as the palm of the hand or larger, which is then dried, and often curiously ornamented and preserved, and highly valued as a trophy by the returning victors. The scalping is an operation not calculated of itself to take life, as it only removes the skin, without injuring the bone of the head. A genuine scalp must contain and show the crown or whirl of the head to prevent that two or more scalps from one head are taken. Besides taking the scalp, the victor generally, if he has time to do it without endangering his own scalp, cuts off and brings home the rest of the hair which the women will divide into a great many small scalp locks, and with them fringe off the seams of shirts and leggings.[23]

Not only were enemies shot with arrows and scalped, they might also be further mutilated. Lewis and Clark encountered tribes west of the Rocky Mountains who took physical trophies other than scalps from their enemies, including jaws, hands, ears, eyes, and fingers, especially "those used to release arrows from the bow."[24] One of the enduring myths of the American frontier is that Geronimo had a necklace of fingers that he treasured and wore into battle against the Chiricahuas' enemies, Indian and non-Indian.

An enemy need not be dead from his arrow wounds to be scalped, and he might even recover from the scalping, depending on his general state of health and the seriousness of his other wounds. Specific medical treatments for scalping were few. More often, treatment was combined with remedies for head wounds. William Thompson, an employee of the Union Pacific Rail Road Company, was scalped by Cheyennes near Plum Creek Station, Nebraska, on August 6, 1867. Thirty-six hours afterward he was seen by Dr. R. C. Moore, who found the scalp entirely removed from a space measuring nine inches long and seven inches wide. The denuded surface extended from one inch above the left eyebrow backward. Thompson also had a severe tomahawk wound on his head. The only dressing Dr. Moore used on the head was surgeons' lint saturated with pure olive oil. In about three weeks the bare outer skull began to separate and ooze pus, but there was no sign of infection in the brain itself. The only pain Thompson experienced was a severe neuralgia down the right side of his head and face, and that ceased after the external bone of the skull peeled and shed. About three months later, scar tissue formed over the entire surface of the skull.[25]

William Thompson was a very lucky man. The usual complications that followed scalping were massive bleeding, infection, and death of the bone, if not of the injured individual as well. The infection was generally localized in the skin and neighboring tissues, but sometimes it became generalized and the patient died from septicemia or meningitis. Necrosis of the skull was always a danger and occasionally didn't appear for several years after the initial injury. When that occurred, the outer portion of the skull became dry and black before it rotted away. When the decay reached the inner bones of the head, an opening into the brain cavity formed and the brain matter popped out. Clearly, the patient's life would then be in extreme danger, even though he might have recovered from his other wounds.

All this brings us back to the early frontier surgeons who, under enormous handicaps, treated the arrow wounds and other afflictions of their men. In cases of serious head injuries the doctors had little hope: the most likely outcome was known well in advance. Nonetheless, the surgeons fought bravely to save lives, using every technique known to medicine and inventing new ones when the old ones didn't serve.

Life-and-death medical struggles still occur all across the land, but now the fight takes place in modern hospitals. Today, highly educated and skillful surgeons stand shoulder to shoulder with the spirits of the battlefield surgeons, the barber-surgeons, and the traditional healers who forged the trail to this high-tech, sophisticated era of modern medicine. Let us not forget them in our race to the twenty-first century and the medical miracles sure to be produced there.

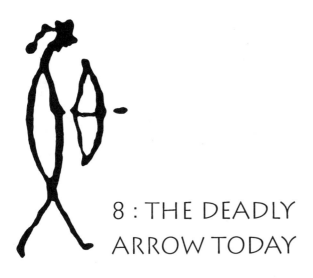

8 : THE DEADLY ARROW TODAY

Efficient in construction and even beautiful when created by artisans, arrows were once terrible weapons of doom and death. They still may be, when abused. Arrow injuries were extremely painful—that is, if death wasn't instantaneous. And the infection that usually followed was often lethal if the wound itself was not. In the 1700s, 1800s, and early 1900s, when the American frontier was still a frontier, there were no "miracle cures," no antibiotics to attack and fight the infection, and no easy ways back to health. Nonetheless, many Native Americans and army personnel recuperated from their injuries and returned to the battle, probably terrified that they would be hurt again. Rightfully so.

The use of bow and arrows today is limited for the most part, one hopes, to hunters in the field, who stalk their wildlife prey as diligently as Native Americans of old pursued their enemies. Modern archery involves mathematical concepts of trajectory, curve, distance, arrow speed, kinetic energy, and charts and graphs on arrow flight.[1] According to an article in *Outdoor Life*, *consistency* = *accuracy* is the equation for a perfect flight formula.[2] Although a great deal of effort has gone into determining the proper weight for arrows, the results have generally been "good news/bad news." Heavy arrows tend to make less noise than lighter arrows, but the latter "pack less wallop," and "decelerate faster"; on the other hand, "the lighter the arrow, the greater the bow noise." My goodness. The Archery Manufacturer's Organization has drawn up a chart that lists safe minimum arrow weights: "The mean safe level was found to be 6 grains of arrow weight per pound of draw weight for a 60 pound cam bow at 30 inch draw length, or, for that bow, 360 grains (6 grains x 60 pounds = 360 grains),"[3] reports an article published in *Sports Afield*.

Other topics of great contemporary interest are the weight of the shafts (superlights are growing in popularity) and the bowstring (Dacron has been the material of choice for years, but other products are beginning to compete). Distance shooting has been charted by "kill and ranging windows measured in yards," resulting in a "kill zone" that equals an eight-inch circle, roughly the size of a deer's vital area. The "kill window" is the difference between the maximum and minimum distances from which your arrows will hit the kill zone. A "ranging window" is the average accuracy with which a person can judge distance to a target. "As long as kill window exceeds ranging window, odds for a killing hit are good."[4]

It certainly would be easy to look at these sophisticated computations and wonder how in the world American Indians of old, without all these high-tech measurements at their disposal, ever shot an arrow and hit a mark. But I won't do that. There is nothing to be accomplished by comparing today's sophistication with a less complicated people and period of American history. Instead, I call your attention to another bowman, a marksman also prominent in mythology whose skill with a bow and arrow is celebrated once a year. This archer is sought after, sung to, welcomed with open arms, dreamed about, symbolized, written about, and practically venerated.

Cupid.

Who wouldn't want to be wounded by one of his arrows?

NOTES

Introduction

1. Smart, "Notes on the 'Tonto' Apaches," p. 418.

2. Holmes, "Manufacture of Stone Arrow Points," p. 49.

3. Grossman, "The Pima Indians of Arizona," p. 414.

4. Mildred Cleghorn, chairperson of the Fort Sill Chiricahua/Warm Springs Apache tribe in Oklahoma, believes that "about 45 percent of the truth has been told about Geronimo in the media. White society is getting closer, slowly, to an understanding of the man" (personal conversations with the author, May 1–5, 1994). Mrs. Cleghorn's group includes relatives of Geronimo, as does the Chiricahua Apache group located on the Mescalero Apache Reservation in south-central New Mexico.

5. The late Eve Ball portrayed the Apache experience from the Chiricahuas' point of view in her book *Indeh: An Apache Odyssey*. Ms. Ball spent nearly thirty years recording information told to her directly by Chiricahua Apaches living on the Mescalero Apache Reservation. Her informants were the sons and daughters of great chiefs and warriors, and they were often themselves survivors of warfare. Ms. Ball loved to tell the story of how difficult it was to get her manuscript published. She was told by various presses that no one was interested in Indians and that while her work was worthy, it wouldn't sell. Finally, Brigham Young University Press took a chance and published *Indeh*. Today it is a classic in its field and one of the few books that document the oral history of the Chiricahua people from their own point of view. Ms. Ball's papers have been donated to the Brigham Young University Library. For information, contact Special Collections and Manuscripts, Harold B. Lee Library, Brigham Young University, Provo, UT 84602. My book *Women of the Apache Nation: Voices of Truth* records Chiricahua oral history as told to me by several elders of the tribe. The book contains interviews with Elbys Naiche Hugar, the great-granddaughter of Cochise, Kathleen Smith Kanseah, Mildred Imach Cleghorn (born a prisoner of war in 1910), and Ruey Haozous Darrow. My *Survival of the Spirit: Chiricahua Apaches in Captivity* addresses the medical catastrophes that befell the Chiricahuas during their nearly thirty years as prisoners of war in Florida, Alabama, and Oklahoma. Interviews with Allan Houser and Berle Kanseah, both descendants of warriors in Mangas Coloradas's and Geronimo's group, and all the interviews in *Women of the Apache Nation* record the experiences of the Chiricahua Apaches from inside the culture.

6. Hoffman, "Poisoned Arrows," pp. 67–70, 74. Hoffman said that "the Scythians, according to Aristotle, prepared their arrow poison by mixing serpent venom with the serum of putrid blood" (p. 67). He also said that Ponce de Leon was fatally wounded by a poisoned arrow while he was searching for the Fountain of Youth (p. 68). On the other hand, Captain John G. Bourke, an army officer who spent a great deal of time observing the Chiricahuas, wrote in 1891 that he did "not believe in the virulence, or rather

in the permanence of the virulence, of the poison made from the putrid liver of deer into which an enraged rattlesnake had ejected its venom" ("Remarks," p. 74). According to Hoffman, the Apaches smeared "a mixture said to consist of decomposed deer liver and rattlesnake venom . . . crushed red ants, centipedes, and scorpions." Hoffman claimed that an examination of the coating on an Apache arrowhead showed the presence of "blood corpuscles and a crystalline substance apparently identical with viperine or crotaline, the acting principle of *Crotalus* venom." He had heard of a wound that began as "a mere scratch upon the upper portion of the scapula, but previous to death the flesh fell from the back as far down as the nates, exposing at various points the ribs and spinal processes." Hoffman went on to say that the Lipan Apaches believed that the poisoned points also possessed "a mystic power" (p. 69). Rattlesnake venom was apparently the poison of choice, and Hoffman listed the Blackfoot, Blood, Piegan, Shoshoni, and Bannock as tribes that used poison on their arrowheads. The Pit River Indians of California, he claimed, used a "dog's liver mixed with the juice of the wild parsnip" (p. 70). Most of the tribes that dipped their arrowheads in poison did so to the accompaniment of chanting, incantations, and other rituals believed to ensure the maximum effect on the enemy.

7. T. Kroeber, *Ishi.*

8. Pope, *Hunting with the Bow & Arrow*, pp. 14–28, 29–37, 46–48, 112–13, 118–19, 242–43, 255.

9. Heizer and Kroeber, *Ishi, the Last Yahi*, p. 176.

10. Ibid., p. 181.

11. Ibid., p. 186.

12. Pope, *Hunting with the Bow & Arrow*, p. 28.

13. Ibid., pp. 118–19, 243, 255.

Chapter 1 : Perspectives

1. McEwen et al., "Early Bow Design and Construction," p. 76.

2. Ibid., p. 80.

3. Bill, "Sabre and Bayonet Wounds," p. 103.

4. The Amerind Museum in Dragoon, Arizona, houses a sample of Geronimo's bows and arrows, which are masterpieces of craftsmanship. Whether these were actually used in warfare or were made by him for the tourist trade is irrelevant from the perspective of an artisan. Carved all along the inner aspect of the bow is a scene complete with tipis and clouds and red dots burned and painted into the tipi walls. Perhaps the dots acknowledge the tribe's early battles with contagious diseases like measles or smallpox. Geronimo's arrows are unpainted and have iron points. Iron-tipped arrows were unknown before contact with Europeans.

5. *Los Angeles Times*, December 14, 1986.

6. *Albuquerque Journal*, May 6, 1993.

7. *Albuquerque Journal*, April 19, 22, 23, 24, 1986.

8. *Albuquerque Journal*, May 8, 1993. The previous record for longest trajectory was recorded in 1798. The Ottoman emperor Sultan Selim III shot two flight arrows 880 meters (about 972 yards), a feat never equaled with archery tackle made using traditional designs.

Chapter 2 : Arrows, Arrow Medicine, and Medicine Arrows

1. Perrone et al., *Medicine Women*, pp. 9–10.

2. Stockel, *Women of the Apache Nation*, pp. 2–3.

3. Ibid., p. 1.

4. Perrone et al., *Medicine Women*, p. 57.

5. Barrett, *Geronimo*, pp. 59–64.

6. Sturtevant, "Seminole Myths of the Origin of Races," pp. 80–81.

7. Morgan, "Human Wolves among the Navaho," pp. 9–10. The Navajos are among the most populous tribes in the United States today. Their name for themselves, Dine, means "the people." According to John Upton Terrell's *American Indian Almanac*, the Navajos believe that they passed through four underworlds until they reached the surface of the earth. "Their Origin Myths relate that most of them were created somewhere in the mountains of southern Colorado. Other Dineh emerged into life somewhere beside the western sea. And all of them moved to live together in Dinetah" (p. 44).

8. Ibid., p. 40.

9. Terrell's *American Indian Almanac* states that the Cheyenne originated in Minnesota, moved to North Dakota, and then were driven into the northern Great Plains along the Missouri River. "Their societal organization almost resembled that of Sparta, with requisites of strict obedience and enormous courage. War was the main goal of the men while the women participated in buffalo hunts and helped the men in other ways" (p. 474). Clearly, this is not a Cheyenne creation myth.

10. *Albuquerque Tribune*, March 12, 1993.

11. Heizer, "An Inquiry into the Status of the Santa Barbara Spear-Thrower," p. 137. The article identifies this instrument as the "Chumash" spear and says it was found in the Santa Barbara area of California.

12. Massey, "The Dart-Thrower in California," p. 57.

13. Massey, "Survival of the Dart-Thrower," p. 91.

14. "Relación," *Documentos Ineditos*, 9:35.

15. Massey, "Survival of the Dart-Thrower," pp. 84–85. Needless to say, Europeans had a valid frame of reference because of their own knowledge of bows and arrows.

16. Rozaire, "A Complete Serrano Arrow," p. 8. Although no exact date could be applied to the specimen, arrows generally replaced atlatl darts after the end of the Basketmaker period, circa 700 A.D. Educated estimates indicate that the Serrano arrow was no more than a few hundred years old when it was found.

17. Ibid., pp. 9–11.

18. Heizer, "How Accurate Were the California Indians?" p. 109.

19. Worcester, "The Weapons of American Indians," p. 228.

20. Ibid., p. 229.

21. Ibid., p. 233.

22. Broadhead, "Elliott Coues and the Apaches," p. 90. John G. Bourke, an army officer and ethnologist who was very familiar with Chiricahua Apache warfare, differed from Coues regarding the Apaches' use of poison (see quotation in Introduction, note 6). He added, "At least I can say that I have seen men and animals struck by darts alleged to have been

so poisoned, but could not perceive that any extra harm had been done thereby" (Bourke, "Remarks," p. 74). Dr. W. J. Hoffman, also writing about Apaches and poisoned arrows, attributed an individual's toxic reaction after being struck by a "poisoned" arrow to septicemia; see Hoffman, "Poisoned Arrows," p. 67.

23. Perry, *Apache Reservation*, p. 100.

24. Ibid., p. 83.

25. I. T. Kelly, "Chemehuevi Shamanism," pp. 137–38. Olbrechts, in "Some Notes on Cherokee Treatment of Disease," discussed black arrowheads used to treat certain ailments such as sore joints. The arrowheads were held against the aching area by the shaman, who sang or recited a time-honored incantation while the "magic" of the arrowhead alleviated the pain. Arrowheads were also used for traditional purposes before battle. The Creeks scratched warriors' arms with arrowheads to enable them to "hold the bow well." In other tribes, men's faces, eyes, and wrists were scratched so as "not to miss when shooting with . . . bow and arrow"; see Walter Krickenberg, "Blood-Letting and Bloody Castigation," pp. 26–34.

26. Devereux, "Mental Hygiene of the American Indian," p. 76.

27. Social stability within a group experiencing intense change is often precarious. The healer holds an exalted position during times of peace, and it is natural for the people to look to him or her when disruption occurs. If the healer is unable to call on his or her power to treat the consequences of the newly introduced agent, the entire group may become unsettled and vulnerable.

28. Townsend, "Disease and the Indian," p. 479.

29. Blish, "The Ceremony of the Sacred Bow," pp. 183–84.

30. C. Kelly, "Arrows from the Rainbow," p. 9.

31. Gatschet, "Medicine Arrows of the Oregon Indians," p. 112.

32. Ottaway, "A Possible Origin for the Cheyenne Sacred Arrow Complex," pp. 94–95.

33. Powell, *Sweet Medicine*, p. 33.

34. This entire tale was related by Peter J. Powell, a Catholic priest who became a close friend of the Cheyenne. He wrote about them from inside their culture, quite a difficult task for a non-Indian. The story about the Cheyenne and the Pawnee was related to Powell by members of the tribe and recorded verbatim. Other versions exist as well.

35. Dorsey, "How the Pawnee Captured the Cheyenne Medicine Arrows," p. 646.

36. Ibid., p. 650.

Chapter 3 : Barbers, Basins, and Battlefields

1. Talbot, "The Early Army Surgeon," p. 336.

2. Wehrli, "The Barber-Surgeon's Shop," p. 272.

3. Will, "The Medical and Surgical Practice of the Lewis and Clark Expedition," pp. 275–76. Under the heading "Physical history and medicine," Rush asked the following questions:

1. What are the acute diseases of the Indians? Is the billious fever attended with a black vomit?

2. Is apoplexy, palsy, epilepsy, madness, rheum(atic) dis-

ease, goitre known among them?

3. What is the state of life as to longevity? At what age do the women *begin and* cease to menstruate?

4. At what age do they marry? How long do they suckle the children? What is the provision of their children after being weaned?

5. The rate of the pulse as to frequency in the morning, at noon, and at night, before and after eating?

6. What is its state in childhood, adult life, and old age? Is it ever subject to intermissions? The number of strokes counted by the quarter of a minute by glass, and multiplied by four will give its frequency in a minute.

7. What are their remedies?

8. Are artificial discharges of blood ever used among them?

9. In what manner do they induce sweating? Do they ever use voluntary fasting? At what time do they use their baths?

10. What is the diet, manner of cooking, and times of eating among the Indians? How do they preserve their food?

Under "Morals," Dr. Rush asked: "(1) What are their vices? (2) Is suicide common among them? Ever from love? (3) Do they employ any substitute for ardent spirits to promote intoxication?

(4) Is murder common among them, and do they punish it with death?" Under "Religion" the questions were "(1) What affinity between their religious ceremonies and those of the Jews? (2) Do they use animal sacrifices in their worship? (3) What are the principal objects of their worship? (4) How do they dispose of their dead, and with what ceremonies do they inter them?" The list is dated May 17, 1803.

4. Ibid., p. 278. These suggestions represent the best remedies for disease prevention and treatment of fatigue, exposure, and cold available in 1803.

5. Sandoz, *The Battle of the Little Big Horn*, p. 35. A copy of this letter, dated July 4, 1876, is in the archives of the Custer Battlefield National Monument, Crow Agency, Montana.

6. McGreevy, "Surgeons at the Little Big Horn," pp. 777–78.

7. *The Old West: The Soldiers*, pp. 218–19. "A Sioux warrior's bow was made of carefully selected ash and strung with two buffalo sinews twisted together . . . the war bow was accurate at over 100 yards—and could be fired more rapidly than muskets or single-shot rifles" (*The Old West: The Indians*, p. 209). Geronimo is believed to have said that the soldiers always gave the Apaches warning because they said, "ready, aim, fire," and by that time the Apaches had scattered (Stockel, *Survival of the Spirit*, p. 251).

8. Wehrli, "Equipment of the First Army Surgeons," pp. 341–42. A bistoury is a long, narrow knife, either straight or curved and sharp-pointed or probe-pointed, designed for cutting from within outward. It was used to open abscesses, enlarge sinuses or fistulas, or cut constrictions in strangulated hernias. A cannula is an artificial tube, of variable size

and shape, usually used for insertion into a body cavity such as an artery or the trachea. These descriptions of the bistoury and cannula are from *Blakiston's Gould Medical Dictionary*, 4th ed.

9. The following information about Dr. Weisel and his work at Fort Davis is from Clary, "The Role of the Army Surgeon in the West."

10. Ibid., pp. 56, 60–64.

11. Utley, *A Clash of Cultures*, p. 32.

12. Ibid., p. 33. Fort Bowie was abandoned in 1894, eight years after the Chiricahua Apaches were taken out of the Southwest as prisoners of war. The general history of the fort is well described by Utley in this document.

13. Nye, *Carbine & Lance*, p. 288. A graphic illustration of a "Comanche postcard" decorates the cover of this book. It shows a soldier looking over his shoulder at an arrow sticking up from his pack, which had been placed on the saddle just behind him. The arrow had just missed the soldier's buttocks.

Chapter 4 : An Explorer-Surgeon Surnamed "Cow's Head"

1. Thompson, "Sagittectomy," p. 1405.

2. In New Mexico this name has been abbreviated to "C de Baca." There are many New Mexicans with that last name.

3. Favata and Fernandez, *Alvar Núñez Cabeza de Vaca's Relación*, p. 12. After his safe return to Spain in 1537, Cabeza de Vaca went on several other expeditions. On November 2, 1541, he set out with 250 men and 26 horses for Asunción, Paraguay, arriving on March 11, 1542. Two years later he left Paraguay in search of the mythical kingdom of El Dorado, but disease and a lack of provisions brought an abrupt halt to the mission. He and his fellow travelers returned to Asunción on April 8, 1544, two weeks before a revolt broke out that resulted in his arrest. He was returned to Seville in chains and later banished from the Americas. His wife expended all her property to defend his honor. Cabeza de Vaca is believed to have died in Seville around 1557. See Thrapp, *Encyclopedia of Frontier Biography*, 1:208.

4. Ibid., p. 55. These may have been the Karankawa Indians, who lived in the coastal area of Texas. The tribe is now extinct.

5. Thompson, "Sagittectomy," p. 1404.

6. Favata and Fernandez, *Alvar Núñez Cabeza de Vaca's Relación*, p. 79.

7. Thompson thought that "psychotherapy for psychosomatic illnesses among a superstitious people could explain most of the results" and that although "Cabeza de Vaca did not have a medical diploma, he was obviously quite enterprising and did what had to be done with the tools at hand, whether by psychotherapy or surgical therapy" ("Sagittectomy," p. 1405).

8. Peckham, *Prehistoric Weapons in the Southwest*.

9. Courville, "Cranial Injuries among the Early Indians of California," p. 184. Courville described the spears as having "shorter handles" and usually "projected with the aid of the atlatl or throwing stick. These were used by the Indians of Florida, Mexico, and of Southwestern America as well as by the Eskimos (these chiefly as harpoons). Perhaps again these throwing spears were chiefly used in hunting, but it is very likely that, as in Mexico, they were also utilized in combat when the occasion demanded"

(p. 185).

10. Ellsworth, *Bows and Arrows*, p. 7.

11. Hodge, *Handbook of American Indians North of Mexico*, p. 92. Widely honored as the patriarch of American Indian studies, Hodge was born October 28, 1864, in Plymouth, England. He came to the United States at age 7, grew up in Washington, D.C., and was educated at the school that became George Washington University. Hodge was John Wesley Powell's stenographer, field secretary to the Hemenway southwestern archaeology expedition, editor of the *American Anthropologist* and various other scholarly journals, executive officer of the Smithsonian Institution, and ethnologist in charge of the Bureau of American Ethnology. He joined the Museum of the American Indian in New York City after he resigned from federal service in 1918. In 1932, at age 67, Hodge became director of the Southwest Museum at Los Angeles, where he served for twenty-two years. He wrote and edited many, many publications. Hodge died in Santa Fe on September 28, 1956, a month short of his ninety-second birthday. See Thrapp, *Encyclopedia of Frontier Biography*, 2:666.

12. Mason, "North American Bows, Arrows, and Quivers," p. 664. This author apparently had private correspondence with Bourke because in a letter Bourke also described feathers used by other tribes and their placements on the shafts.

13. Mason, "Amerindian Arrow Feathering," p. 584.

14. Pope, *Bows and Arrows*, p. 48.

15. Hamilton, *Native American Bows*, p. 4.

16. Rt. Rev. Robert S. Ove, letter to the author, February 1993. One of Geronimo's bows is housed in the Amerind Museum in Dragoon, Arizona. It is a magnificent piece of work, complete with a scene etched into its belly by the warrior himself showing a line of tipis, clouds, and rain. When Geronimo was a prisoner of war, he was taken by the American government to several world's fairs and expositions. At the St. Louis World's Fair in 1904, the old man sold his handmade bows and arrows from a very popular private booth at the Louisiana Purchase Exposition. It is not known whether the bow now in the Amerind Museum was sold to a member of the public at that time. Although he was still incarcerated, Geronimo was permitted to keep any profits he made from his craftwork. He was so famous during the latter years of his confinement (the Apaches were imprisoned from 1886 to 1914) that buttons sold right off his jacket and his printed autograph brought twenty-five cents, a goodly sum at the time.

17. Hamilton, *Native American Bows*, p. 11.

18. Ibid., p. 58.

19. Courville, "Cranial Injuries among the Early Indians of California," p. 183.

20. Laubin and Laubin, *American Indian Archery*, p. 16. The authors emphasized Apache bows and arrows because of that tribe's presence in the Southwest when Cabeza de Vaca roamed the area. The Apache presence in the area dates back to 1525, just a few years before the Spaniards arrived (Stockel, *Survival of the Spirit*). An Athapascan group, the Apaches had other names for themselves. Supposedly they were dubbed *Apachu* ("enemy" in the Zuni language) by the Zuni Puebloans, a peaceful people living in villages on high mesas in Arizona. It is not unreasonable to conclude that the

arrowhead removed by Cabeza de Vaca from an Indian's chest was shot by a member of an Apache band or that he was among the Pueblo Indians at the time the operation took place. Unfortunately, accurate identification of the host tribe is difficult, if not impossible.

21. Mason, "North American Bows, Arrows, and Quivers," pp. 668–69.

22. Laubin and Laubin, *American Indian Archery*, p. 28.

23. Thanks to Dan L. Thrapp for this information. Thrapp himself timed an expert flint knapper, a white man. Using only materials that would have been available to a Native American eleven thousand years ago, including a bit of elk antler for a hammer, the knapper started with a block of stone and created a perfect Folsom point in twenty minutes flat, and did not appear to hurry doing it.

24. Peckham, *Prehistoric Weapons*.

25. Bill, "Notes on Arrow Wounds," p. 368.

26. DaCosta, *Modern Surgery*, pp. 302–03.

27. Russell, *Indian Artifacts*, p. 131. "Baking" could have been accomplished in aboriginal pit ovens.

28. Ewers, "Self-torture in the Blood Indian Sun Dance," p. 168. This article describes a Plains Indian sun dance in which an iron arrowhead was used to pierce a warrior's chest before a serviceberry stick was inserted through each breast. The man's back was also cut open with an arrowhead and skewers were inserted into the wounds. Ewers recorded first-person experiences of three young men of the Blood tribe who participated in a sun dance in 1889. For anyone unfamiliar with the sun dance, I recommend this article as an introduction.

29. Honea, *Early Man Projectile Points in the Southwest*. Most of the information about southwestern points in this chapter is from this work.

30. Thanks to Towana Spivey for this tidbit, which he relayed in a conversation on July 28, 1993.

31. This is my opinion; others may not agree. The truth is probably somewhere between the two points of view.

Chapter 5 : Be All That You Can Be in the Ar-r-r-mee, circa 1860

1. Bill, "Sabre and Bayonet Wounds," p. 103.

2. Rogers, "The Aboriginal Bow and Arrow," p. 266. For a tabular presentation of the function of the fingers and thumb in the various forms of arrow release, see A. L. Kroeber, *Arrow Release Distributions*.

3. Bill, "Sabre and Bayonet Wounds," p. 109.

4. Wilson, "Arrow Wounds," p. 531.

5. Bill, "Notes on Arrow Wounds," p. 369.

6. *Surgeon General's Report*, p. 145.

7. Ibid., p. 155.

8. The arrows used by Navajos and Utes were about two and a half feet long. Apache, Comanche, Arapaho, Cheyenne, Kiowa, and Pawnee arrows were about three inches longer.

9. Bill, "Notes on Arrow Wounds," p. 368.

10. Bill, "Sabre and Bayonet Wounds," p. 118.

11. *Surgeon General's Report*, p. 155.

12. Wilson, "Arrow Wounds," p. 527.

13. Ibid., p. 524.

14. Bill, "Notes on Arrow Wounds," p. 384. How the pressure created by a

block or a pile of books actually helped the physician to remove the offending object was not made clear, but it probably gave him a better leverage base for extracting arrows embedded in bone.

15. Collodion was a dressing routinely used for battlefield wounds. It was made by dissolving pyroxylin (a product obtained by mixing nitric and sulfuric acids on cotton; also known as soluble guncotton) in ether and alcohol. According to Robert Druitt's *Principles and Practices of Modern Surgery*, p. 138, collodion is a useful substitute for adhesive plaster. It dries instantly, forming a film that adheres firmly and forms an artificial scab. When applied between sutures it prevents air from reaching damaged tissue. The book suggests holding the edges of the wound together and applying a single thick layer of collodion to the wound.

16. Wilson, "Arrow Wounds," p. 525.

17. Ibid., p. 530. The use of a silk handkerchief as a buffer to ease the journey of the shaft through the body may seem surprising, but the treatment of battlefield wounds in the 1800s produced many innovative practices designed to save lives. Unfortunately, many have since been lost.

18. Frederick McAninch, Arizona Historical Society, telephone conversation with the author, July 24, 1993, and undated letter mailed July 29, 1993; Arizona State Museum, Human Identification Laboratory, letter dated January 21, 1990, to Department of Transportation and Flood Control regarding AZ BB:13:9, Burials 1 and 2. Special thanks to Fred McAninch for this information.

19. *Surgeon General's Report*, p. 163.

20. Mason, "North American Bows, Arrows, and Quivers," pp. 665–66.

21. Bill, "Sabre and Bayonet Wounds,"

p. 116. Conrad died in 955 B.C.

22. Bill, "Notes on Arrow Wounds," p. 385.

23. Thrapp, *Encyclopedia of Frontier Biography*, 3:1452; and Thrapp, *Conquest of Apacheria*, pp. 36–37.

24. Bill, "Sabre and Bayonet Wounds," p. 108.

Chapter 6 : The Mother of All Headaches

1. Courville, "Cranial Injuries among the Early Indians of California," p. 194.

2. Ibid., p. 195.

3. Ibid., p. 203.

4. Ibid., p. 204.

5. Ibid., p. 196.

6. Bill, "Sabre and Bayonet Wounds," pp. 115–16.

7. Army Medical Museum, Path. Series no. 6677.

8. *Surgeon General's Report*, p. 146. Descriptions of arrow wounds to all areas of the body form the bulk of the information in this very interesting report. Many case histories contain substantial details about particular wounds and their treatment. Postmortem data are occasionally provided.

9. *Grumous* means "granular" or "grainy."

10. Bill, "Sabre and Bayonet Wounds," pp. 111–12.

11. Bill, "Notes on Arrow Wounds," p. 374.

12. Ibid., p. 375.

13. *Surgeon General's Report*, pp. 147–48.

14. Ibid., pp. 149–50. Included with the description is a woodcut of the skull of Private Martin W— showing the arrowhead embedded in his head. The soldier's

last name was not given.

15. Ibid. A temperature chart of this man, known only as JC, accompanies the case history.

16. Aconite is a very poisonous drug obtained from the roots of *Aconitum napellus* (monkshood). It has a bitter, pungent taste and leaves a sensation of numbness and tingling on the lips and tongue. Physiologically, it is a cardiac, respiratory, and circulatory depressant, and it produces sensory paralysis. The principal alkaloid present is aconitine. It has been used as a diaphoretic, antipyretic, and diuretic (*Blakiston's Gould Medical Dictionary*, p. 17).

17. Bill, "Sabre and Bayonet Wounds," p. 115. If the wounded man couldn't reach a physician quickly, or if the physician couldn't locate the missile in the patient's head, Dr. Bill advised that "the case must be left altogether to nature."

18. Courville, "Cranial Injuries among the Early Indians of California," p. 150. Dan Thrapp interviewed Cyril Courville in 1957. Courville was born February 19, 1900, and died on March 22, 1968. He was a physician and the managing editor of the *Bulletin of the Los Angeles Neurological Society*. Much of his research was devoted to the study of cranial injuries among North American and early California Indians. He collected weaponry designed for skull-assaulting purposes as well as skulls and photos of skulls exhibiting the effects of flint weaponry, war clubs, tomahawks, and bludgeoning implements of all kinds. His publications include photographs of skulls with flint points—arrowheads, spear points, or atlatl projectiles—deeply buried in them and bone growing about the incision, plainly indicating that the victims survived the impact (Thrapp, *Encyclopedia*

of Frontier Biography, 4:115–16; the encyclopedia contains many interesting entries about the people on the American frontier).

19. Courville, "Cranial Injuries among the Early Indians of California," p. 160.

Chapter 7 : The Head: Cutting, Scraping, Drilling, and Scalping

1. Most Native Americans knew natural remedies for stopping bleeding. For example, Percival ("Primitive Treatment of Disease," pp. 330–31) reported that if the wound was caused by a bite, the native licked it and went to a nearby stream to wash it with cold water. If the bleeding continued or if the wound was more severe, the individual pressed the edges together with his fingers and tied leaves over the injury until he could get back to camp and have it attended to by tribal members more skilled in treating injuries. Such treatments, both in camp and away, were tried and trusted methods. Often the treatment included songs and incantations designed to encourage healing. These varied from tribe to tribe, but the actual natural remedies could be similar in a region. I was once told by an Apache woman that she stopped superficial bleeding by applying spiderwebs to the cut after she pressed its edges together. She had been out in the desert hunting for herbs when she lost her balance and fell into a thorny cactus that sliced open a segment of her outer upper arm. While it was bleeding she looked for and found a spiderweb nearby and applied it gently to the cut. The bleeding stopped, and she returned to her home to have the wound cleaned and treated. She showed me the small scar that re-

mained. Fortunately, spiderwebs know no particular geography. On the other hand, medicinal plants that grow in the desert Southwest, for example, are not found in the Great Plains, meaning that there is regional variation in the plant medicines preferred by Native Americans.

2. Clarke et al., *A Century of American Medicine*, p. 170.

3. Rogers, "Trephined Skulls," p. 1.

4. Freeman, "Surgery of the Ancient Inhabitants of the Americas," p. 23. Stramonium is derived from the dried leaves and flowering tops of the datura plant, which contains the alkaloids hyoscyamine and scopolamine. It is similar to belladonna in its actions.

5. "By trepanation, in the modern sense," reported Aleš Hrdlička, "is meant a surgical operation in life on the head and skull, the object of which is either to relieve pressure on the brain by an indented portion of the vault, or to reach and cure some pathological condition on or in the brain" ("Trepanation among Prehistoric People"). Hrdlička's reference to "modern sense" contains no parameters, but he went on to state that "perforations of the skull of the dead . . . were practiced in different parts of the world since Neolithic times . . . the practice of trephining in the Old World originated in Europe and northern Africa apparently during the time of the megalithic constructions, five thousand to four thousand years ago." Hrdlička, who studied skulls that had been trephined, was at the time—and in my opinion still is—the foremost expert on the subject of paleopathology.

6. Moes, "Medicines of the California Indians," p. 4.

7. Stewart, "Stone Age Skull Surgery," p. 481.

8. Cosgrove, "A Note on a Trephined Indian Skull from Georgia," p. 356.

9. According to Wakefield and Dellinger ("Possible Reasons for Trephining the Skull in the Past," p. 166), "primitive man regarded disease as belonging to one of three categories: 1. Disease was something projected into the body of the victim. 2. Disease was something which could be taken from the body of the victim. 3. Disease was the effect of something on some part of, or some object connected with, the body of the victim." They concluded that "it is reasonable . . . to state that whenever and wherever the first human skull was trephined, probably one of these concepts, or more than one, was the compelling motive for the procedure. The operation was performed: (1) to permit the entry or projection of something into the body of the victim, (2) to permit escape of, or to take from the body, something, or (3) to combat sorcery."

10. Lumholtz and Hrdlička, "Trephining in Mexico," p. 390. Lumholtz explored Tarahumara country and discovered the skulls, and Hrdlička examined them and offered his expert opinion on the trephining each skull had undergone.

11. Freeman, "Primitive Surgery," p. 445.

12. Hrdlička, "Trepanation among Prehistoric People," pp. 173, 175.

13. Shapiro, "Primitive Surgery," p. 266.

14. Rogers, "Healing of Trephine Wounds," p. 326. About scraping, Hrdlička said, "An extensive scraping, down to the inner compact layer and perhaps even through this in spots, would cover several square inches of the forehead, or of

the top of the cranium. When the opening was through, the edges of the bone were smoothed or beveled" (quoted in Rogers, ibid., p. 327).

15. Ibid., pp. 327–29.

16. Freeman, "Primitive Surgery," p. 445. In this same article a medicine man is described as an individual "of more than ordinary tact, knowledge and intellect" who, with "fantastic dances and gestures, facial contortions and weird chantings exercised a hypnotic influence on his patients, leading to relaxation and sleep." Freeman first delivered this paper as a presidential address before the Western Surgical Association in Omaha, Nebraska, on December 14, 1917.

17. Hrdlička, "Disease, Medicine and Surgery," p. 1664. Thrapp's *Encyclopedia of Frontier Biography* (2:686–87) identifies Hrdlička as an anthropologist born in Humpolec, Bohemia, on March 29, 1869. He emigrated to the United States with his father in 1882 and earned medical degrees. In 1903 he "joined the National Museum of the Smithsonian Institution where he built up one of the world's largest human skeletal collections." Hrdlička's special interest was the variation in body measurements seen in different populations. Hrdlička wrote widely, particularly about Native Americans. He died in Washington, D.C., on September 5, 1943.

18. Shapiro, "Primitive Surgery," p. 266.

19. *Albuquerque Journal*, July 19, 1993.

20. Nadeau, "Indian Scalping," pp. 180, 184.

21. Ackerknecht, "Head Trophies in America," p. 1670.

22. Reese, "History of Scalping," pp. 327–31. The article cites other references regarding scalping throughout history, but there is no bibliography and the author did not identify his immediate sources. Nonetheless, this article is an excellent depiction of scalping from prehistory forward.

The J. Wesley Powell mentioned is the same ethnologist who explored the Grand Canyon from May through August 1869. He made the journey again in 1871 and conducted other explorations in Arizona and Utah in 1874 and 1875, after which he became director of the federal survey of the Rocky Mountain region in 1875. Powell became director of the Bureau of American Ethnology (BAE) in 1879 and held that position until his death on September 23, 1902. While at the BAE, he also became director of the U.S. Geological Survey in 1881, heading it until his retirement in 1894 (Thrapp, *Encyclopedia of Frontier Biography*, 3:1169).

23. Reese, "History of Scalping," pp. 331, 333. The lack of specificity with regard to tribe is troublesome. For example, Catlin said all North American Indians scalped, which is certainly not true. And not all warriors brought home the scalps to their women for recycling as fringe. The fearsome Chiricahua Apaches were repulsed by the idea of scalping, even though some of their actions against their enemies, Indian and non-Indian, might be considered a good deal more brutal than scalping.

24. Ibid., p. 337.

25. Ibid., pp. 340–41.

Chapter 8 : The Deadly Arrow Today

1. "Taming Trajectory," p. 32.

2. Adams, "Perfect Flight Formula,"
p. 20.

3. Schuh, "Lighter Arrows," p. 38.

4. Schuh, "Distance Shooting," p. 50.

Glossary

1. These entries were selected from the "Vocabulary of Archery" in Mason, "North American Bows, Arrows, and Quivers," pp. 635–36.

GLOSSARY
OF BOW AND ARROW
TERMINOLOGY[1]

Arm-guard. A guard worn on the outer side of the forearm to catch the blow of the string.

Arrow. A piercing, stunning, or cutting missile shot from a bow.

Arrow cement. A substance used to fasten the arrowhead to the shaft. A few tribes used glue or cement to make sinew-backed bows.

Arrowhead. The part of an arrow designed to produce a wound. The parts of the primitive stone arrowhead are the tip, or apex; the faces; the sides, or edges; the base, shank, or tang; and the facettes.

Back. The part of the bow away from the archer.

Backed. A bow is said to be backed when strips of wood, bone, horn, rawhide, baleen, sinew, or cord are fastened along the outside to increase the elasticity.

Base (of an arrowhead). The portion that fits into the shaft.

Belly. The part of a bow facing the archer.

Bow. An elastic weapon for casting an arrow from a string. It is the manual part of the weapon.

Bow arm. The arm that holds the bow.

Bow case. A long bag or case of wood, skin, leather, or cloth in which the bow is kept when not in use. Same as quiver.

Bow shot. The distance an arrow flies when released from a bow.

Bow stave. The bow in a rough state. Bow staves were important items of commerce before guns came on the scene, and every thrifty Indian kept several on hand to work on at his leisure.

Bowstring. The string used in discharging a bow. The substances used to make the string and the methods of treatment and nocking are important characters.

Bow wood. The substances used for bows; generally wood, but horn, antler, bone, and metal were also employed.

Bowyer. A maker of bows. In many tribes bow making was considered a profession.

Bracer. A wrist guard or other contrivance for protecting the archer's wrist from being galled by his bowstring.

Bracing. Stringing or bending the bow and putting the eye of the string over the upper nock preparatory to shooting.

Built-up bow. A bow made by gluing pieces of elastic wood and other substances together, as in Asiatic examples.

Chipping hammer. Also called a hammer stone, this is a stone used for knocking off chips, or spalls, in making stone arrowheads. There are really two kinds: the hammer stone and the chipping hammer.

Cock-feather. The feather of an arrow that is uppermost when the bow is drawn.

Compound bow. A bow made of two or more pieces of wood, bone, antler, horn, or whalebone lashed or riveted or spliced together.

Eye. The loop of a bowstring that passes over the upper nock in bracing.

Faces. The broad, flat portions of an arrowhead.

Facettes. The little surfaces left by chipping out a stone arrowhead.

Feathering. The strips of feather at the butt of an arrow.

Flaker. The pointed implement of bone, antler, etc., used to shape flint arrowheads, spearheads, etc., by pressure.

Footing. A piece of wood inserted in the shaftment of an arrow at the nock.

Foreshaft. A piece of hard wood, bone, ivory, antler, etc., at the front tip of an arrow that gives it extra weight and serves as a site of attachment for the head or movable barb.

Grafted bow. A species of compound bow formed of two pieces joined together at the handle or grip.

Grip. The part of a bow that is grasped in the hand.

Horns. The ends of a bow, also called ears.

Limbs. The parts of a bow above and below the handle or grip.

Nock. Properly, the notch in the horn of the bow, but applied also to the whole of that part on which the string is fastened. The upper nock is the one held upward in bracing, and the lower nock is placed on the ground. Also, the notched part in the end of an arrow.

Nocking. Placing the arrow on the string preparatory to shooting.

Nocking point. The place on a bowstring where the nock of the arrow is to be fitted.

Noose. The end of a string that occupies the lower horn of a bow.

Packing. The substance used in binding the nocks and the grip of bows.

Pile. The head of an archery arrow.

Quiver. A case for holding the weapons of the archer.

Reinforcements. Splints of a rigid material built into a compound or sinew-backed bow.

Release. Letting go the bowstring in shooting.

Riband. A term applied to the stripes painted on arrow shafts, generally around the shaftment. These ribands are also called clan marks, owner marks, game tallies, etc.

Self-bow. A bow made of a single piece of wood or other material.

Shaft. The portion behind the head of an arrow.

Shaft grooves. Furrows cut along an arrow shaft from the head backward.

Shaftment. The part of an arrow on which the feathering is laid.

Shank. The part of an arrowhead corresponding to the tang of a sword blade.

Sides (of an arrowhead). The sharpened portions between the apex and the base, also called the edges.

Sinew-backed bow. A bow whose elasticity is increased by the use of sinew along the back. The sinew is applied either in a cable, as among the Eskimo, or in a layer attached by means of glue, as in the western United States.

Spall. A large flake of stone knocked off in blocking out arrowheads.

Stele. The wooden part of an arrow; an arrow without feathers or head.

Stringer. A maker of bowstrings.

Tip. The sharp apex of an arrowhead.

Veneer. A thin strip of tough, elastic substance glued to the back of a bow.

Weight (of a bow). The number of pounds required to draw a bow until the arrow may stand between the string and the belly.

BIBLIOGRAPHY

Ackerknecht, Erwin H. "Head Trophies in America." *Ciba Symposia* 5 (1944): 1670–76.

Adams, Chuck. "Perfect Flight Formula." *Outdoor Life* (October 1993):20.

Ball, Eve. *Indeh: An Apache Odyssey*. Provo: Brigham Young University Press, 1980.

Barrett, S. M. *Geronimo: His Own Story*. New York: Ballantine Books, 1970.

Bill, J. H. "Notes on Arrow Wounds." *American Journal of Medical Science* 44 (1862):365–87.

———. "Sabre and Bayonet Wounds; Arrow Wounds." In *International Encyclopedia of Surgery*, vol. 2, ed. John Ashhurst, Jr. New York: William Wood & Company, 1881–86.

Blakiston's Gould Medical Dictionary. 4th ed., ed. A. R. Gennaro et al. New York: McGraw-Hill, 1979.

Blish, Helen H. "The Ceremony of the Sacred Bow of the Oglala Dakota." *American Anthropologist*, n.s., 36 (1934):180–87.

Bourke, John G. [Captain, U.S. Army]. "Remarks." *American Anthropologist* 4 (1891):71–74.

Broadhead, Michael J. "Elliott Coues and the Apaches." *Journal of Arizona History* 14, no. 2 (1973):87–94.

Clarke, Edward H., Henry J. Bigelow, Samuel D. Gross, T. Gaillard Thomas, and J. S. Billings. *A Century of American Medicine 1776-1876*. 1876. Reprint. New York: Lenox Hill, 1971.

Clary, David A. "The Role of the Army Surgeon in the West: Daniel Weisel at Fort Davis, Texas, 1868–1872." *Western Historical Quarterly* 3, no. 1 (1972):53–66.

Cosgrove, C. B. "A Note on a Trephined Indian Skull from Georgia." *American Journal of Physical Anthropology* 13, no. 2 (1929):353–57.

Courville, Cyril B. "Cranial Injuries among the Early Indians of California." *Bulletin of the Los Angeles Neurological Society* 17, no. 4 (1952):137–62.

———. "Cranial Injuries among the Indians of North America." *Bulletin of the Los Angeles Neurological Society* 13, no. 4 (1948):181–219.

DaCosta, John C. *Modern Surgery*. 8th ed. Philadelphia: W. B. Saunders, 1919.

Devereux, G. "The Mental Hygiene of the American Indian." *Mental Hygiene* 26 (1942):71–84.

Dorsey, George A. "How the Pawnee Captured the Cheyenne Medicine Arrows." *American Anthropologist*, n.s., 5 (1903):644–58.

Druitt, Robert. *The Principles and Practices of Modern Surgery*. Philadelphia: Henry C. Lea, 1867.

Ellsworth, Clarence. *Bows and Arrows*. Los Angeles: Southwest Museum Leaflets, 1950.

Ewers, John C. "Self-torture in the Blood Indian Sun Dance." *Journal of the Washington Academy of Sciences* 38, no. 5 (1948):166–73.

Favata, Martin A., and José B. Fernandez, trans. *The Account: Alvar Núñez Cabeza de Vaca's Relación*. Houston: Arte Público Press, 1993.

Freeman, Leonard M. "Primitive Surgery of the Western Hemisphere." *Journal of the American Medical Association* 70

(1918):443–48.

———. "Surgery of the Ancient Inhabitants of the Americas." *Art and Archeology* 18 (1924):21–36.

Gatschet, Albert S. "Medicine Arrows of the Oregon Indians." *Journal of American Folk-Lore* 6 (1893):111–12.

Grossman, F. E. [Captain, U.S. Army]. "The Pima Indians of Arizona." In *Smithsonian Institution Annual Report for 1871*, pp. 407–19. Washington, D.C.: Smithsonian Institution Press, 1873.

Hamilton, T. N. *Native American Bows*. York, Pa.: George Shumway, 1972.

Hamm, Jim. *Bows and Arrows of the Native Americans: A Complete Step-by-Step Guide to Wooden Bows*. New York: Lyons and Burford, 1991.

Heizer, Robert F. "How Accurate Were the California Indians with the Bow and Arrow?" *Masterkey* 44 (1970): 108–11.

———. "An Inquiry into the Status of the Santa Barbara Spear-Thrower." *American Antiquity* 4 (1938):137–41.

———. "Introduced Spearthrowers (Atlatls) in California." *Masterkey* 19 (1945):109–12.

Heizer, Robert F., and Theodora Kroeber. *Ishi, the Last Yahi: A Documentary History*. Berkeley: University of California Press, 1979.

Hodge, Frederick W. *Handbook of American Indians North of Mexico*. New York: Rowman and Littlefield, 1971.

Hoffman, W. J. "Poisoned Arrows." *American Anthropologist* 4 (1891): 67–71.

Holmes, W. H. "Manufacture of Stone Arrow Points." *American Anthropologist* 4 (1891):49–58.

Honea, Kenneth. *Early Man Projectile Points in the Southwest*. Popular Series Pamphlet no. 4. Santa Fe: Museum of New Mexico Press, 1976.

Hrdlička, Aleš. "Disease, Medicine and Surgery among the American Aborigines." *Journal of the American Medical Association* 99 (1932):1661–66.

———. "Trepanation among Prehistoric People, Especially in America." *Ciba Symposia* 1 (1939):170–77.

Kelly, Charles. "Arrows from the Rainbow." *Desert Magazine* 7, no. 11 (1944):9–11.

Kelly, Isabel T. "Chemehuevi Shamanism." In *Essays in Anthropology*, ed. Robert H. Lowie, pp. 129–42. Berkeley: University of California Press, 1936.

Krickenberg, Walter. "Blood-letting and Bloody Castigation among the American Indians." *Ciba Symposia* 1 (1939):26–34.

Kroeber, A. L. *Arrow Release Distributions*. University of California Publications in American Archeology and Ethnology 23, no. 4 (1927):283–96.

Kroeber, Theodora. *Ishi in Two Worlds*. Berkeley: University of California Press, 1961.

Laubin, Reginald, and Gladys Laubin. *American Indian Archery*. Norman: University of Oklahoma Press, 1980.

Lumholtz, Carl, and Aleš Hrdlička. "Trephining in Mexico." *American Anthropologist* 10, no. 12 (1897):389–96.

Mason, O. "Amerindian Arrow Feathering." *American Anthropologist* 1 (1899):583–85.

———. "North American Bows, Arrows, and Quivers." In *Smithsonian Institution Annual Report for 1893*, pp. 631–79. Washington, D.C.: Smithsonian Institution Press, 1894.

Massey, William. "The Dart-Thrower in Baja California." *Davidson Journal of*

Anthropology 3 (1957):55–62.

———. "The Survival of the Dart-Thrower on the Peninsula of Baja California." *Southwestern Journal of Anthropology* 17 (1961):81–93.

McEwen, Edward, Robert L. Miller, and Christopher A. Bergman. "Early Bow Design and Construction." *Scientific American* 264 (June 1991):76–83.

McGreevy, Patrick S. "Surgeons at the Little Big Horn." *Surgery, Gynecology & Obstetrics* 140 (May 1975):774–80.

Moes, Robert J. "Medicines of the California Indians." *Branding Iron* (Spring 1993):4. Los Angeles Westerners Corral No. 191.

Morgan, William. "Human Wolves among the Navajo." *Yale University Publications in Anthropology* 11 (1936):3–43.

Nadeau, Gabriel. "Indian Scalping: Technique in Different Tribes." *Bulletin of the History of Medicine* 10 (1941):178–94.

Nye, W. S. *Carbine & Lance: The Story of Old Fort Sill*. Norman: University of Oklahoma Press, 1988.

Olbrechts, F. "Some Notes on Cherokee Treatment of Disease." *Janus* 33 (1928):271–80.

The Old West: The Indians. New York: Time-Life Books, 1973.

The Old West: The Soldiers. Alexandria, Va.: Time-Life Books, 1974.

Ottaway, Harold N. "A Possible Origin for the Cheyenne Sacred Arrow Complex." *Plains Anthropologist* 15 (1970):94–98.

Peckham, Stewart. *Prehistoric Weapons in the Southwest*. Popular Series Pamphlet no. 3. Santa Fe: Museum of New Mexico Press, 1965.

Percival, J. Barkley. "Primitive Treatment of Disease." *Medical Record* 93 (1918):330–31.

Perrone, Bobette, H. Henrietta Stockel, and Victoria Krueger. *Medicine Women, Curanderas, and Women Doctors*. Norman: University of Oklahoma Press, 1989.

Perry, Richard J. *Apache Reservation: Indigenous Peoples & the American State*. Austin: University of Texas Press, 1993.

Pope, Saxton T. *Bows and Arrows*. 1923. Reprint. Berkeley: University of California Press, 1974.

———. *Hunting with the Bow & Arrow*. New York: G. P. Putnam's Sons, 1925.

Porter, Joseph C. *Paper Medicine Man: John Gregory Bourke and His American West*. Norman: University of Oklahoma Press, 1986.

Powell, Peter J. *Sweet Medicine: The Continuing Role of the Sacred Arrows, the Sun Dance, and the Sacred Buffalo Hat in Northern Cheyenne History*. Vol. 1. Norman: University of Oklahoma Press, 1969.

Reese, Hans H. "The History of Scalping and Its Clinical Aspects." *Yearbook of Neurology* (1940):325–41.

"Relación del descubrimiento del reino de California por el capitán y cabo Nicholas de Cardona." In *Documentos Ineditos relativos el descubrimientos . . . America y Oceania*, vol. 9. Madrid, 1862–1900.

Rogers, Spencer L. "The Aboriginal Bow and Arrow of North America and Eastern Asia." *American Anthropologist* 42 (1940):155–69.

———. "Healing of Trephine Wounds." *American Journal of Physical Anthropology* 23, no. 3 (1938):321–39.

———. "Trephined Skulls." Slide Set 1. San Diego Museum of Man, 1980.

Rozaire, Charles. "A Complete Serrano Arrow." *Masterkey* 36 (1962):8–14.

Russell, Virgil Y. *Indian Artifacts*. Boulder, Colo.: Johnson Publishing, 1962.

Sandoz, Mari. *The Battle of the Little Big Horn*. Philadelphia and New York: J. B. Lippincott, 1966.

Schuh, Dwight. "Distance Shooting." *Sports Afield* (September 1993):50.

———. "Lighter Arrows—Good News, Bad News." *Sports Afield* (January 1993):38.

Shapiro, H. L. "Primitive Surgery: First Evidence of Trephining in the Southwest." *Natural History* 27 (1927): 266–69.

Smart, Charles [Brevet Captain and Assistant Surgeon, U.S. Army]. "Notes on the 'Tonto' Apaches." In *Smithsonian Institution Annual Report for 1867*, pp. 417–19. Washington, D.C.: Smithsonian Institution Press, 1868.

Stewart, T. D. "Stone Age Skull Surgery: A General Review with Emphasis on the New World." In *Smithsonian Institution Annual Report for 1957*, pp. 469–91. Washington, D.C.: Smithsonian Institution Press, 1958.

Stockel, H. Henrietta. *Survival of the Spirit: Chiricahua Apaches in Captivity*. Reno: University of Nevada Press, 1993.

———. *Women of the Apache Nation: Voices of Truth*. Reno: University of Nevada Press, 1991.

Sturtevant, William C. "Seminole Myths of the Origin of Races." *Ethnohistory* 10 (1963):80–86.

Surgeon General's Office. *A Report of Surgical Cases Treated in the Army of the United States from 1865 to 1871*. Washington, D.C.: Government Printing Office, 1871.

Talbot, L. "The Early Army Surgeon." *Ciba Symposia* 1 (1940):334–39.

"Taming Trajectory." *Field and Stream* (November 1993):32.

Terrell, John Upton. *American Indian Almanac: The Authoritative Reference and Chronicle*. New York: Thomas Y. Crowell, 1974.

Thompson, Jesse E. "Sagittectomy— First Recorded Surgical Procedure in the American Southwest, 1535: The Journey and Ministrations of Alvar Núñez Cabeza de Vaca." *New England Journal of Medicine 289*, no. 26 (1973):1403–07.

Thrapp, Dan L. *The Conquest of Apacheria*. Norman: University of Oklahoma Press, 1967.

———. *Encyclopedia of Frontier Biography*. 4 vols. Glendale, Calif.: Arthur H. Clark, 1988. Paperback, 4 vols. Lincoln: University of Nebraska Press, 1991.

Townsend, James G. "Disease and the Indian." *Scientific Monthly* 47 (December 1938):479–95.

Utley, Robert M. *A Clash of Cultures: Fort Bowie and the Chiricahua Apaches*. Department of the Interior, National Park Service. Washington, D.C.: Government Printing Office, 1977.

Wakefield, E. G., and Samuel Dellinger. "Possible Reasons for Trephining the Skull in the Past." *Ciba Symposia* 1 (1939):166–69.

Wehrli, G. A. "The Barber-Surgeon's Shop." *Ciba Symposia* 1 (1939):270–74.

———. "Equipment of the First Army Surgeons." *Ciba Symposia* 1 (1940): 341–43.

Will, Drake W. "The Medical and Surgical Practice of the Lewis and Clark Expedition." *Journal of the History of Medicine* (July 1959):273–97.

Wilson, Thomas. "Arrow Wounds."

American Anthropologist 3 (1901):
513–31.

Worcester, D. E. "The Weapons of American Indians." *New Mexico Historical Review* 20 (1945):227–38.

INDEX

K

Kilbourne, H. S. (U.S. Army physician), 69

Kiowas, 68. *See also* Satamore

Kirkman, Jason, 4

Klamath Lake Indians: healing ceremony of, 21

Knight, C. W. (U.S. Army physician), 85

Kroeber, Theodora, xvi

L

Laubin, Reginald and Gladys, 50–52

Legends and myths: Alaskan, 77; Cheyenne, 11, 78; Chiricahua Apache, 8; concerning construction materials of arrowheads, 57; concerning Geronimo's necklace of fingers, 99; Iroquois, 77; Navajo, 10–11; Pawnee, 22–27

Lumholtz, Carl, 91

M

Mason, Otis T., 46

Massey, William, 13

McAninch, Frederick, 71

McEwen, Edward, 1–2

Medicine, Native American: remedies, traditional, 112n. 1;
—societies: Arrow Keepers, Cheyenne, 23; Sacred Bow Society, Oglala Dakota, 19

Middleton, P. (U.S. Army physician), 65

Miller, Robert L., 1–2

Modoc Indians: healing ceremony of, 21

Moes, Robert, 89

Mohave Indians: and cure of gunshot wounds, 18

Mooney, James, 97

Moore, R. C., 99–100

N

Native American peoples: Alaskan, 77; Apaches, 45, 48–52; Aravaipa Apaches, xi–xiii; Chemehuevi, 17; Cherokee, 106n. 25; Cheyenne, 11, 21–27, 78, 99, 105n. 9; Chiricahua Apaches, 3, 8, 16, 36, 103nn. 4, 5, 6, 105–6n. 22, 109n. 20, 112n. 1, 114n. 23; Chumash, 85; Cocopa, 18; Comanche, 2, 16, 70–71, 84; Creeks, 106n. 25; Crow, 18; Eskimo, 46; Hopi, 54; Iroquois, 77; Kiowas, 68–69; Klamath Lake, 20; Modoc, 20; Mohave, 18; Navajo, 10–11, 67, 74, 105n. 7; Oglala Dakota, 19; Paiute, 20, 54; Pawnee, 16, 23–27, 68–69, 78; Pima, xiii; Plains, 78, 110n. 28; Pueblos of New Mexico and Arizona, 15, 95; Salishan, 46; Seminole, 8–10; Shasta, 14; Sioux, 2, 32, 79, 107n. 19; Tonto Apaches, xi–xii; Ute, 82; Yahi, xiv, xviii; Yuma, 18

Navajos: creation myth of, 105n. 7; and death from arrow wounds, 67

Notson, W. M. (U.S. Army physician), 84

O

Ottaway, Harold, 23

P

Pawnee Indians: and Cheyennes, 23–27; and Kiowas, 68; use of atlatls and lances by, 16. *See also* Kiowas; Satamore

Pima Indians, xiii

Peabody, J. H. (U.S. Army physician), 69

Peckham, Stewart, 41–42, 45, 48, 52

Perry, Richard J., 16–17

Points. *See* Arrowheads

Poison arrowheads, xiv; Apache, Chiricahua, 16; and application of poison to arrowhead, 54; described by

Poison arrowheads (*continued*)
Bourke, 103–104n. 6, 105n. 22; described by W. J. Hoffman, 103n. 6; Hopi, 54; Paiute, 54; reaction of body to, 63, 66. *See also* Infections
Pope, Saxton, xv, xviii, 48
Powell, J. Wesley, 114n. 22
Pueblo Indians of New Mexico: trephining by, 95; weapons of, 15

Q

Quivers: construction and materials of, 52

R

Reese, Hans H., 97, 99
Rekate, Harold, 96
Roberts, Anthony, 3–4
Rogers, Spencer L., 62–63, 94–95
Rush, Benjamin, 31, 32, 106–7n. 2
Russell, Virgil Y., 54–55

S

Sacred Bow Society of Oglala Dakota, 19, 20
Salishan tribes, 48
Satamore (Kiowa chief), 68–69
Scalping: cultural endorsement of, 97; history of, 97; technique of, 99; treatment of, 97–100
Seminole Indians: creation myth of, 8, 10
Shamanism: Chemehuevi, 17; Klamath Lake and Modoc, 21; Mohave, 18
Shapiro, Harry L., 94
Shasta Indians: skill of, in shooting arrows, 14
Skull, surgery on: and bone regeneration, 96; and shamans, 89; South American indigenous peoples' techniques for, 88, 95; use of amulets in, 90. *See also* Trephining
Skull collections: American Museum of Natural History, 95; Harvard University, 95; Lima, Peru, 95; San Diego Museum, 96; United States National Museum, 95
Soto, Hernando de, 14
Spivey, Towana, 57
Stewart, T. D., 90
Stramonium: use of, in treatment of arrow wounds, 113n. 4
Surgeons, barber and military: battlefield equipment of, 33, 63–64, 107n. 8; professional history of, 29–31
Sweet Medicine (Cheyenne culture hero), 22–27

T

Thompson, Jesse, 41
Thompson, William, 99–100
Thrapp, Dan L., 75, 112n. 18; on Aleš Hrdlička, 114n. 17
Trephining: ante-mortem, 90; described by Hrdlička, 113nn. 5, 14; implements used for, 89, 94; methods of, 94–95; post-mortem, 90; by Pueblo Indians of New Mexico, 95; reasons for, 89–91, 113n. 9; survival rate after, 95. *See also* Skull, surgery on

U

U.S. Army physicians: J. H. Bill, 3, 54, 62–75, 80–81, 82–83, 85; A. T. Comfort, 72; Elliott Coues, 16; W. H. Forwood, 69; C. C. Gray, 80; H. S. Kilbourne, 69; C. W. Knight, 85; P. Middleton, 65; C. W. Notson, 85; J. H. Peabody, 69; Charles Smart, 83–84; Daniel Wiesel, 34–35; H. C. Yarrow, 85
Utley, Robert, 36

V

Vaca, Alvar Núñez Cabeza de, 37–41, 108n. 3. *See also* Explorers and Writers, Spanish

W

White Painted Woman (Chiricahua
  Apache deity), 8
Wiesel, Daniel (U.S. Army physician),
  34–35. *See also* Fort Davis, Texas
Worcester, D. E., 16
Wounds, arrow. *See* Arrowheads, treat-
  ment of wounds from
Wounds, head, 87, 99. *See also* Scalping

Y

Yahi Indians: arrowheads of, xvii; arrows
  of, xvi–xvii; bows of, xv; quivers of,
  xviii. *See also* Ishi
Yarrow, H. D. (U.S. Army physician), 85
Yuma Indians, 18